Fundamentals of Bile Duct Injuries

Juan Pekolj • Victoria Ardiles • Juan Glinka
Editors

Fundamentals of Bile Duct Injuries

From Prevention to Multidisciplinary Management

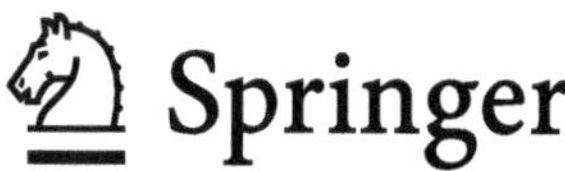

Editors
Juan Pekolj
General Surgery Service & Liver Transplant Unit
Buenos Aires, Buenos Aires, Argentina

Victoria Ardiles
General Surgery & Liver Transplant Unit
Hospital Italiano de Buenos Aires
Buenos Aires, Buenos Aires, Argentina

Juan Glinka
HPB Surgery; Multi-Organ Transplantation
Western University
London, ON, Canada

ISBN 978-3-031-13385-5 ISBN 978-3-031-13383-1 (eBook)
https://doi.org/10.1007/978-3-031-13383-1

This Springer imprint is published by the registered company Springer Nature Switzerland AG
The registered company address is: Gewerbestrasse 11, 6330 Cham, Switzerland

To all the previous members of the HPB Surgery Section of the General Surgery Service of Hospital Italiano de Buenos Aires Argentina

To my mentors Dr. Enrique Marcelo Beveraggi and Dr. Eduardo de Santibañes

To my daughters Tatiana, Milenka, and Ivana, my anchor in the life.

Juan Pekolj

To my husband, Arturo, and my children, Felipe, Francisco, and Emilia.

To my mentor, Dr. Eduardo de Santibañes for his permanent guidance, inspiration, and support.

Victoria Ardiles

In memory of my beloved mother, Odilia.

To the apple of my eyes, Florencia and Carmela.

My little "warrior hearts" brothers, Vladimir and Jeremias.

To Eduardo de Santibañes, Ernesto Molmenti and Ephraim Tang for their permanent support and inspiration.

And to the co-editors Juan Pekolj and Victoria Ardiles for the immense privilege of working with them in this project.

Juan Glinka

Epilogue

Bile duct injuries (BDI) are still an important complication of cholecystectomy, either open or laparoscopic. Nowadays, after 35 years from the first laparoscopic cholecystectomy, BDI are still the Achille's heel of this approach.

BDI is a topic of great concern for surgeons, due to the life risk and unpredictable results on the patient, and the potential litigation with the physical and mental consequences for the surgeon ("second victim").

The consensus about the management of a BDI, must be done in a referent center by means of a multidisciplinary approach. The spectrum of treatment for these patients is so wide, from a percutaneous abdominal drainage to a liver transplantation, and in the middle of multiple different options.

The Section of Hepato-Pancreato-Biliary (HPB) Surgery, in the General Surgery Service from the Hospital Italiano de Buenos Aires in Argentina was created in the year 1974. Since that moment, the team was a referent group in the country and in South America for the management of BDI. Also, we perform close to 700 LC per year, and this allows us, with our own BDI, to understand the mechanism and intraoperative diagnose and propose algorithms for the management in this crucial moment. Our section is very well trained in BDI repair, liver resection, and liver transplantation.

Our hospital also has a very developed Image Service, Gastroenterology and Endoscopy Service, Critical Care Service, and a Biliary Multidisciplinary Team, making our institution as an ideal place for treating BDI.

The objective of this book is to give a simple and useful publication, easy to apply in daily activities, and to publish our experience in the different topics of the management of BDI.

Our thanks go to all the chapter authors for their time and dedication giving clear messages and to our General Surgery Service and its members and our Hospital

Italiano de Buenos Aires for allowing us to grow without limits. A special thanks go to Springer Editorial for their trust in our project and helping us in the process of developing this book.

Juan Pekolj, MD, PhD
Victoria Ardiles, MD, PhD
Juan Glinka, MD

Contents

Contributors

Guillermo Arbues, MD HPB Surgery, Hospital Italiano de San Justo, San Justo, Argentina

Victoria Ardiles, MD, PhD HPB Surgery and Liver Transplant Unit, Hospital Italiano de Buenos Aires, Buenos Aires, Argentina

David Alberto Biagiola, MD HPB Surgery and Liver Transplant Unit, Sanatorio Parque, Rosario, Argentina

Eduardo de Santibañes, MD, PhD HPB Surgery and Liver Transplant Unit, Hospital Italiano de Buenos Aires, Buenos Aires, Argentina

Martín de Santibañes, MD, PhD HPB Surgery and Liver Transplant Unit, Hospital Italiano de Buenos Aires, Buenos Aires, Argentina

Ignacio Fuente, MD Upper GI and Bariatric Surgery Unit, General Surgery Service, Hospital Italiano de Buenos Aires, Buenos Aires, Argentina

Juan Glinka, MD Division of HPB Surgery and Multiorgan Transplant Unit, Western University – London Regional Cancer Program, London, ON, Canada

Jeremias Goransky, MD HPB Surgery, Hospital Italiano de San Justo, San Justo, Argentina

Pablo Huespe, MD Image-Guided Minimally Invasive Surgery Unit, Hospital Italiano de Buenos Aires, Buenos Aires, Argentina

Sung Ho Hyon, MD, PhD Image-Guided Minimally Invasive Surgery Unit, Hospital Italiano de Buenos Aires, Buenos Aires, Argentina

Julio C. Lazarte, MD HPB Surgery, Clínica Pasteur, Neuquen, Argentina

Carlos Macías Gómez, MD Gastroenterlogy Department, Hospital Italiano de Buenos Aires, Buenos Aires, Argentina

Federico Marcaccio, MD Páncreas Unit, Sanatorio Las Lomas, Buenos Aires, Argentina

Oscar Mazza, MD HPB Surgery, General Surgery Service, Hospital Italiano de Buenos Aires, Buenos Aires, Argentina

Ignacio Merlo, MD General Surgery Service, Hospital Italiano de Buenos Aires, Buenos Aires, Argentina

Ramiro Orta, MD Body Imaging, HBP Section, Sanatorio Parque, Rosario, Argentina

Martin Palavecino, MD HPB Surgery, General Surgery Service, Hospital Italiano de San Justo, San Justo, Argentina

HPB Surgery, General Surgery Service, Hospital Italiano de San Justo, Prov Buenos Aires, Argentina

Juan Pekolj, MD, PhD General Surgery Service & Liver, Transplant Unit, Buenos Aires, Buenos Aires, Argentina

Rodrigo Sanchez Cláriá, MD HPB Surgery and Intestinal Transplant Unit, Hospital Italiano de Buenos Aires, Buenos Aires, Argentina

Juan Carlos Spina, MD Body Imaging, HBP Section, Hospital Italiano de Buenos Aires, Buenos Aires, Argentina

Marcos Zandomeni, MD General and HPB Surgery, Hospital Durand, Buenos Aires, Argentina

Chapter 1
Introduction

Juan Pekolj

More than 35 years after the first Laparoscopic Cholecystectomy (LC), Bile Duct Injuries (BDI) remains one of the most worrisome complications [1].

It is important to understand that these types of injuries are inherent not only in biliary surgery but also in many abdominal procedures: they have always existed and have always been a major problem. In this context, it should be remembered that, in the USA, the Lahey Clinic was a national referral center for the repair of these complications at the time of Open Cholecystectomy (OC) [2].

The incidence of BDI after LC seems to have decreased, compared to the initial periods, ranging between 0.2% and 0.5% among large systematic reviews carried out in France and the USA. However, the risk of BDI in LC is still deemed 1.79 times higher than in OC [3].

In our hospital series, the rate of BDI in open surgery is 0.19% (12 lesions out of 6266 procedures), while in LC is 0.17% (20 lesions out of 11,423 laparoscopic biliary surgeries) having diagnosed the BDI intraoperatively in more than 90% of cases [4].

The trends in the incidence of BDI among different series can be appreciated in Table 1.1.

This devastating complication represents numerous admissions to specialized Hepatopancreatobiliary (HPB) units, where patients frequently arrive with the sequelae from previously attempted treatments and require more complex procedures such as repeated surgeries, hepatectomies, or eventually liver transplantation (LT) [1].

J. Pekolj (✉)
General Surgery Service & Liver, Transplant Unit, Buenos Aires, Buenos Aires, Argentina
e-mail: juan.pekolj@hospitalitaliano.org.ar

J. Pekolj et al. (eds.), *Fundamentals of Bile Duct Injuries*,
https://doi.org/10.1007/978-3-031-13383-1_1

Table 1.1 Incidence of BDI among different series

Author	Year	n	Incidence (%)
Southern S.C [5]	1991	1518	0,5
Zha Y [6]	2010	13,000	0,08
Giger A [7]	2011	31,838	0,3
Hamad E [8]	2011	2955	0,18
Pekolj J [9]	2013	10,123	0,18
Y. El Dhuwaib [10]	2016	572,223	0,09
Pucher P [11]	2018	505,292	0,32 – 0,52

The risk factors for a BDI can be divided into three groups: dependent on the surgeon (level of training), on the patient (obesity, anatomical variants, acute, and chronic inflammatory processes), and on the institution (equipment, availability of fluoroscopy) [12].

The degree of training in the procedure has been shown to have a close relationship with the injury rate; although the high level of training does not rule out the possibility of injuries since more complex cases are addressed [13].

In the pathogenesis of BDI, the main conditioning mechanisms of injury are (a) Misinterpretation of regional anatomy and (b) Technical errors such as blind hemostatic maneuvers and the misuse of energy devices [14, 15].

The use of Intra Operative Cholangiography (IOC) has served mainly to achieve an intraoperative diagnosis of the situation and to limit the extension of a BDI when it occurred. In this situation, the utilization of IOC is associated with "minors" BDI and thus, amenable to be repaired primarily and without conversion to open surgery in the setting of a LC.

The associated vascular lesions in BDI are conditioning factors of greater severity and the need for more complex treatments such as liver resections and in some cases LT.

The occurrence of a BDI exposes us to a complex scenario, making its evolution and final results always hard to predict, not to mention that the patient's life will always be at risk.

In the event of a diagnosis during surgery, the surgeon is abruptly in a terrible moment to continue operating, therefore in an ideal case scenario, the surgeon should follow the consensual recommendation to call another surgeon for support, or even better, arrange the referral to a specialized center [16].

Repairs of what are considered "minor injuries' have shown great results even in the hands of the surgeon who generated the BDI. However, major injury repairs clearly need to be handled by experienced HPB surgeons within specialized centers [9].

The advancement of laparoscopic skills in modern surgical training, allows intra- and postoperative repairs to be increasingly frequent, having the benefits of Minimally Invasive Surgery (MIS) without compromising the outcomes.

Surgical repairs are accompanied by non-negligible morbidity (26.3%) and mortality of up to 5% in nonelective repair cases. Even the expectancy and quality of life in these patients have been markedly altered. A patient with a BDI has a 10 times increased risk of dying in the first year compared to a patient who underwent cholecystectomy and did not have this complication. Moreover, the patient's life expectancy is decreased by 10 years [17, 18].

Current discussions are focused on prevention, on the selection of the best time of repair, on the optimal technique, who should repair them, on the role of endoscopic and percutaneous procedures, and on long-term outcomes [19] (Fig. 1.1).

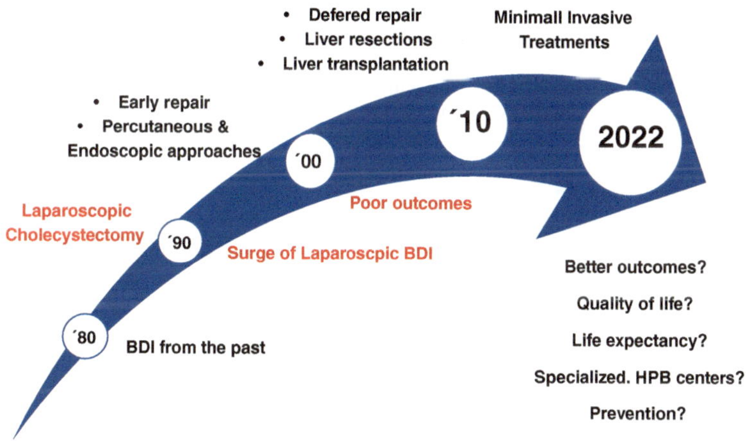

Fig. 1.1 Timeline of the evolution of the various topics related to BDIs and their correlation with the decades in which they were the main topics of discussion

To summarize, the following standards should be pursued in any surgery service: a low incidence of BDI, a high rate of intraoperative diagnosis and eventually treatment, and complex repairs to be performed by surgeons trained in advanced HPB surgery.

References

1. Schreuder AM, Busch OR, Besselink MG, Ignatavicius P, Gulbinas A, Barauskas G, Gouma DJ, van Gulik TM. Long-term impact of iatrogenic bile duct injury. Dig Surg. 2020;37:10–21.
2. Asbun HJ, Rossi RL, Lowell JA, Munson JL. Bile duct injury during laparoscopic cholecystectomy: mechanism of injury, prevention, and management. World J Surg. 1993;17(547–51):551–2.
3. Pesce A, Palmucci S, La Greca G, Puleo S. Iatrogenic bile duct injury: impact and management challenges. Clin Exp Gastroenterol. 2019;12:121–8.
4. de Santibáñes E, Ardiles V, Pekolj J. Complex bile duct injuries: management HPB. 2008;10:4–12.
5. Southern Surgeons Club. A prospective analysis of 1518 laparoscopic cholecystectomies. N Engl J Med. 1991;324:1073–8.
6. Zha Y, Chen X-R, Luo D, Jin Y. The prevention of major bile duct injures in laparoscopic cholecystectomy: the experience with 13,000 patients in a single center. Surg Laparosc Endosc Percutan Tech. 2010;20:378–83.
7. Giger U, Ouaissi M, Schmitz S-FH, Krähenbühl S, Krähenbühl L. Bile duct injury and use of cholangiography during laparoscopic cholecystectomy. Br J Surg. 2011;98:391–6.
8. Hamad MA, Nada AA, Abdel-Atty MY, Kawashti AS. Major biliary complications in 2,714 cases of laparoscopic cholecystectomy without intraoperative cholangiography: a multicenter retrospective study. Surg Endosc. 2011;25:3747–51.
9. Pekolj J, Alvarez FA, Palavecino M, Sánchez Clariá R, Mazza O, de Santibañes E. Intraoperative management and repair of bile duct injuries sustained during 10,123 laparoscopic cholecystectomies in a high-volume referral center. J Am Coll Surg. 2013;216:894–901.
10. El-Dhuwaib Y, Slavin J, Corless DJ, Begaj I, Durkin D, Deakin M. Bile duct reconstruction following laparoscopic cholecystectomy in England. Surg Endosc. 2016;30:3516–25.
11. Pucher PH, Brunt LM, Fanelli RD, Asbun HJ, Aggarwal R. SAGES expert Delphi consensus: critical factors for safe surgical practice in laparoscopic cholecystectomy. Surg Endosc. 2015;29:3074–85.
12. Alvarez FA, de Santibañes M, Palavecino M, Sánchez Clariá R, Mazza O, Arbues G, de Santibañes E, Pekolj J. Impact of routine intraoperative cholangiography during laparoscopic cholecystectomy on bile duct injury. Br J Surg. 2014;101:677–84.
13. Chen CB, Palazzo F, Doane SM, Winter JM, Lavu H, Chojnacki KA, Rosato EL, Yeo CJ, Pucci MJ. Increasing resident utilization and recognition of the critical view of safety during laparoscopic cholecystectomy: a pilot study from an academic medical center. Surg Endosc. 2017;31:1627–35.
14. Conrad C, Wakabayashi G, Asbun HJ, et al. IRCAD recommendation on safe laparoscopic cholecystectomy. J Hepatobiliary Pancreat Sci. 2017;24:603–15.
15. Strasberg SM, Brunt LM. Rationale and use of the critical view of safety in laparoscopic cholecystectomy. J Am Coll Surg. 2010;211:132–8.
16. Strasberg SM, Pucci MJ, Brunt LM, Deziel DJ. Subtotal cholecystectomy-"Fenestrating" vs "reconstituting" subtypes and the prevention of bile duct injury: definition of the optimal procedure in difficult operative conditions. J Am Coll Surg. 2016;222:89–96.

17. Koppatz H, Sallinen V, Mäkisalo H, Nordin A. Outcomes and quality of life after major bile duct injury in long-term follow-up. Surg Endosc. 2021;35:2879–88.
18. Hariharan D, Psaltis E, Scholefield JH, Lobo DN. Quality of life and medico-legal implications following iatrogenic bile duct injuries. World J Surg. 2017;41:90–9.
19. Brunt LM, Deziel DJ, Telem DA, et al. Safe cholecystectomy multi-society practice guideline and state of the art consensus conference on prevention of bile duct injury during cholecystectomy. Ann Surg. 2020;272:3–23.

Chapter 2
Anatomical Considerations

Martín de Santibañes and Eduardo de Santibañes

Introduction

Perfect knowledge of the anatomy of the porta hepatis (PH) and its structures, as well as their relations and variations, is of vital importance for a safe surgery and to avoid navigating the storm of a BDI.

In this chapter, we will provide information on the anatomy and practical tips to avoid misinterpretation of the different landmarks when approaching this always challenging anatomical region.

The Hilar Plate

The Hilar Plate (HP) system consists of bile ducts and blood vessels, which are surrounded by a sheath of connective tissue that is continued by the Glisson's capsule, at the intrahepatic level, and the hepatoduodenal ligament, in its extrahepatic portion (Fig. 2.1). This system also has a large number of lymphatics, nerves, and a vascularized network [1].

Since Couinaud investigations, we know that the bile ducts and the Hepatic Artery (HA) are located within this system, while the Portal Vein (PV) is covered by a separate sheath of a laxer connective tissue, which explains why the vasculo-biliary structures can be easily separated from the PV during its surgical dissection [2].

M. de Santibañes (✉) · E. de Santibañes
HPB Surgery and Liver Transplant Unit, Hospital Italiano de Buenos Aires, Buenos Aires, Argentina
e-mail: martin.desantibanes@hospitalitaliano.org.ar; eduardo.desantibanes@hospitalitaliano.org.ar

J. Pekolj et al. (eds.), *Fundamentals of Bile Duct Injuries*,
https://doi.org/10.1007/978-3-031-13383-1_2

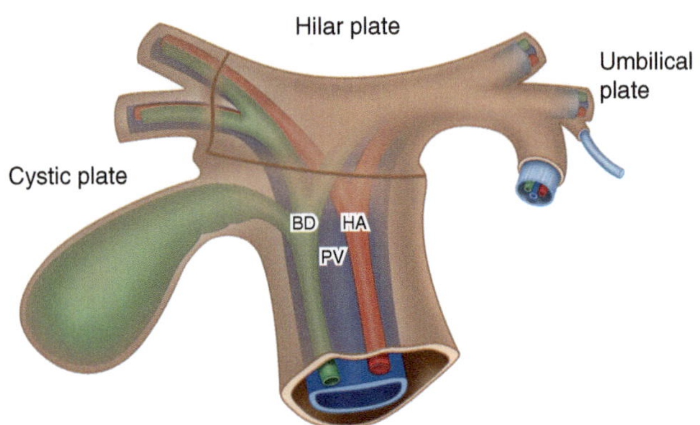

Fig. 2.1 The Hilar Plate (HP). *BD* bile duct, *PV* portal vein, *HA* hepatic artery

Anatomy of the Biliary Tree

The anatomy of the biliary tree follows that of the portal system and the segmentation of the liver. According to the vascular anatomy, the right and left hemi-liver are drained by a right and left hepatic duct, respectively.

Segment I (with its three well-defined portions: the Spiegel segment, the caudate process, and the paracaval portion) is drained by several ducts that join in both rights and left ducts near the posterior side of the biliary confluence at the level of the hepatic triad.

Let's analyze separately the different structures that encompass the biliary system [3].

Main Bile Duct

The Common Hepatic Duct (CHD) typically receives the Cystic Duct (CD), to distally shape the Common Bile Duct (CBD). This distinction is arbitrary, as the CD joins at a variable site and must be carefully considered during gallbladder surgery. The main bile duct runs down and anterior to the PV, joining its left margin at the medial part of the PH [4].

The HA, which runs upward, is usually located on the left of the PH. The right branch of the HA usually runs posterior to the CBD and anterior to the PV.

The CBD forms the left border of "Calot's triangle," which is bounded by the inferior surface of the right lobe of the liver as the upper limit, and by the CD as the lower limit. This is where the cystic artery, one of the elements to be divided during a cholecystectomy, is located [5].

When there is no inflammation in the PH, it is often possible to identify anatomical variations by the transparency of the tissues, without any dissection.

It should always be considered that, when there is a variation in the biliary anatomy, there may be variations in other vascular structures or vice versa.

Biliary Confluence

The biliary confluence or commonly named "Carrefour" is usually extrahepatic. Although it can be lowered down even more upon the dissection of the fibrotic sheath that represents the HP at that level if required for specific surgical procedures.

This biliary confluence normally extends along and anterior to the origin of the right branch of the PV. The duct is displaced superiorly and medially to the left of the main PV.

However, variations are common, and this "classic" disposition occurs only in 60% of cases [6].

Right Hepatic Duct

The Right Hepatic Duct (RHD) is characterized by a small common trunk (1 cm) and typically lies at the right of the PV. This portion in general has an extrahepatic location [7].

Deeper in the liver parenchyma, the right anterior (for segments V and VIII) and the right posterior (for segments VI and VII) hepatic ducts branch off the RHD.

It is worth mentioning when that the right posterior duct typically branches off the RHD posteriorly and from the left ("the north-turning") and less frequently inferiorly and from the right ("the south-turning") [8, 9].

Variations in the entry of the RHD into the CBD make this typical bifurcation disappear and must be considered when planning any liver resection or CBD exploration.

In 15% of cases, there is a "trifurcation" of the hepatic ducts (RHD, RPD, and LHD).

During a cholecystectomy, potential variations of the RPD should be always suspected (Fig. 2.2) as most of these are extrahepatic and easy to injury inadvertently [10].

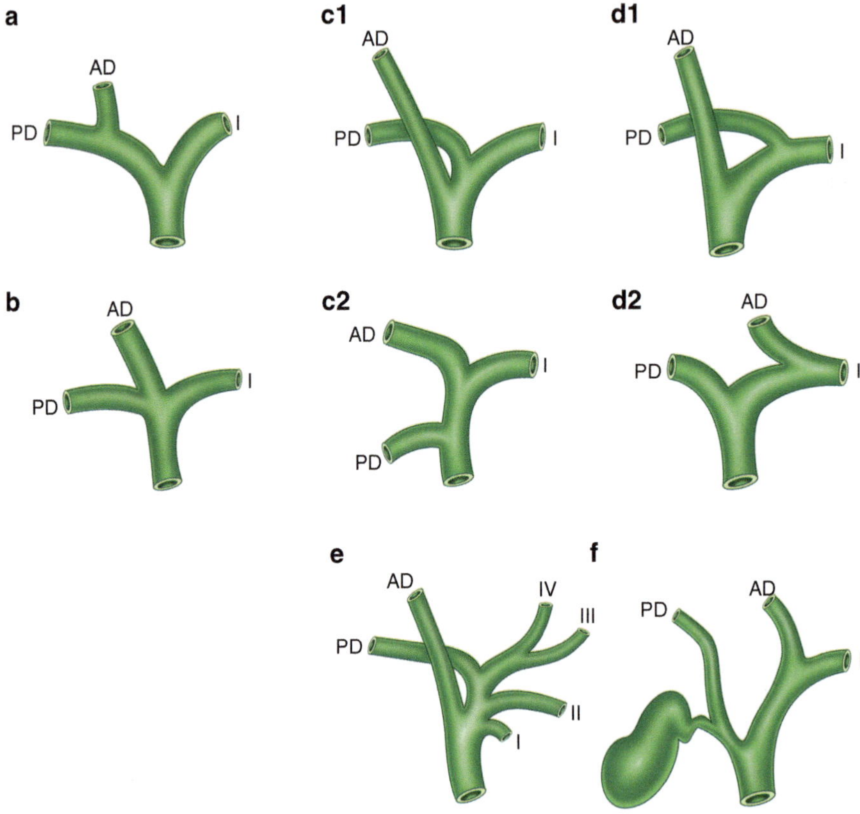

Fig. 2.2 Anatomical variations of the proximal bile duct. *PD* Right Posterior Duct, *AD* Right Anterior Duct, *LD* Left Duct Hepatic Duct segment I, Hepatic Duct Segment II Hepatic Duct Segment III, Hepatic Duct Segment IV

Left Hepatic Duct

The Left Hepatic Duct (LHD) is usually extrahepatic, longer, and more horizontal compared to the RHD. Although sometimes might be vertical and deeply located.

It usually forms a common duct, following the "Rex or Retzius process" distribution, and branches the ducts for segments II, III, and IV of the liver [11].

It is important to bear in mind that the RPD can lead to the LHD on its posterior side (8–26%) and less frequently to the RHD (6–8%).

As this aberrant anatomy is intrahepatic, does not represent a problem for cholecystectomy but does represent a challenge when considering a liver resection.

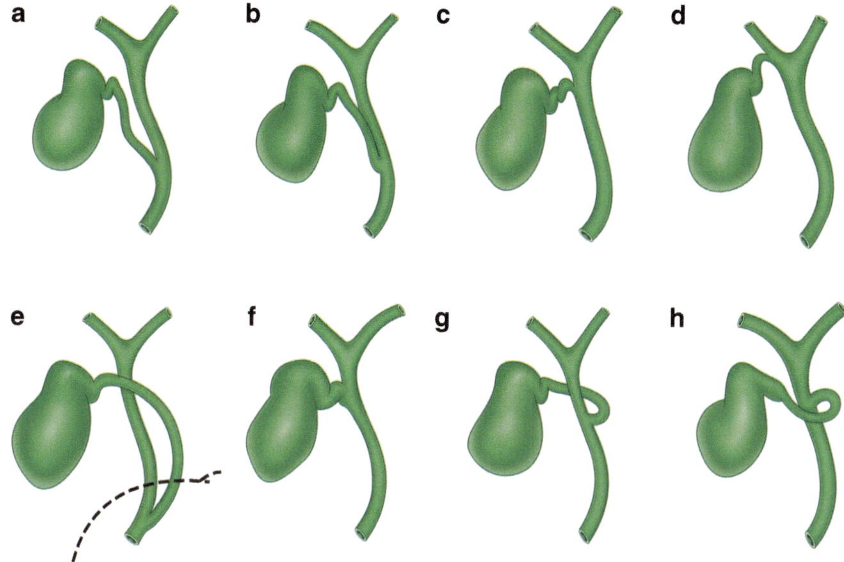

Fig. 2.3 Variations in the relation of the Cystic Duct (CD) to the Common Bile Duct (CBD). (**a**) Low insertion into common hepatic duct. (**b**) Parallel cystic and common hepatic duct. (**c**) High insertion into common hepatic duct (**d**) Cystic duct drains into right hepatic duct. (**e**) Long cystic duct that joins common hepatic duct behind the duodenum. (**f**) Absence of cystic duct. (**g**) Cystic duct crosses posterior to common hepatic duct and joins it anteriorly. (**h**) Cystic duct courses anterior to common hepatic duct and joins it posteriorly

Variations of the Cystic Duct

The Cystic Duct (CD) usually ends into the CBD in an angular (75%), parallel (20%), and spiral form on its left (5%). Given these numerous variations, it is not uncommon to misinterpret the CBD as the CD during a cholecystectomy when they are running really parallel to each other [12].

It is also worth mentioning as well that in 2% of cases, the RPD may lead into the CD or just above it, and thus be misinterpreted as the CD itself [13].

Sometimes the short CD leads to this anatomical variant ultimately serving as a risk factor for BDI (Fig. 2.3).

Subvesical Bile Ducts

The Subvesical Bile Ducts (SBD) or commonly known as "Ducts of Luschka" are represented by small (usually less than 2 mm) accessory bile ducts from the liver draining directly into the gallbladder [14]. There is another widely accepted theory suggesting that they are just subvesical accessory ducts with no real communication with the gallbladder, although they might become evident when surgeons lose the dissection plane during a cholecystectomy. We must highly suspect an SBD injury when we advert bile coming off through the gallbladder fossa and attempt its primary closure once other causes of bile leaks have been ruled out. Their overall prevalence is reported to be around 4%, however, this can be underestimated [15].

Recent studies suggest that about 27% of clinically relevant bile leaks might be caused by an injury or disruption of an SBD [16].

Essential aspects to visualize and interpret the anatomy during a cholecystectomy:

1. Have the necessary instruments for the procedure, with adequate positioning of the trocars and a 30-degree optic.
2. Cephalic traction of the gallbladder fundus and lateral traction (pointing to the patient's right shoulder), to reduce redundancy of the infundibulum.
3. Puncture and evacuation of the gallbladder to improve its retraction, in cases where traction cannot be performed easily (acute cholecystitis) [17].
4. Lateral and caudal traction of the infundibulum, for correct exposure of Calot's triangle, exposing the CD and artery.
5. "Critical view of Safety" to avoid misidentification of the bile ducts, ensuring that only two structures (CD and artery) are attached to the gallbladder. For this, they must be dissected separately, and the proximal third of the gallbladder must be moved from its fossa, to ensure that there is no anatomical variant there [18].
6. Systematic use of intraoperative cholangiography. Ideally by transcystic route or possibly by a puncture of the gallbladder.
7. Ligation of the cystic duct with knots ("endoloop") to prevent migration of metallic clips that could condition a postoperative leak.
8. In case of severe inflammation of the gallbladder pedicle, with its retraction or lack of recognition of cystic structures, a subtotal cholecystectomy might be indicated.
9. In case of hemorrhage, avoid indiscriminate clip placement and or blind cautery. Opt for compressive maneuvers and, once the bleeding site has been identified, evaluate the best method of hemostasis.
10. If the surgeon is not able to resolve the injury caused, it is always better to ask for help from a colleague, and if necessary, to refer the patient to a specialized center.

References

1. Roskams T, Desmet V. Embryology of extra- and intrahepatic bile ducts, the ductal plate. Anat Rec. 2008;291:628–35.
2. Abou-Khalil JE, Bertens KA. Embryology, anatomy, and imaging of the biliary tree. Surg Clin North Am. 2019;99:163–74.

3. Charels K, Klöppel G. The bile duct system and its anatomical variations. Endoscopy. 1989;21(Suppl 1):300–8.
4. Larobina M, Nottle PD. Extrahepatic biliary anatomy at laparoscopic cholecystectomy: is aberrant anatomy important? ANZ J Surg. 2005;75:392–5.
5. Abdalla S, Pierre S, Ellis H. Calot's triangle. Clin Anat. 2013;26:493–501.
6. Takeishi K, Shirabe K, Yoshida Y, et al. Correlation between portal vein anatomy and bile duct variation in 407 living liver donors. Am J Transplant. 2015;15:155–60.
7. Chaib E, Kanas AF, Galvão FHF, D'Albuquerque LAC. Bile duct confluence: anatomic variations and its classification. Surg Radiol Anat. 2014;36:105–9.
8. Vakili K, Pomfret EA. Biliary anatomy and embryology. Surg Clin North Am. 2008;88(1159–74):vii.
9. Kafle A, Adhikari B, Shrestha R, Ranjit N. Anatomic variations of the right hepatic duct: results and surgical implications from a cadaveric study. J Nepal Health Res Counc. 2019;17:90–3.
10. Catalano OA, Singh AH, Uppot RN, Hahn PF, Ferrone CR, Sahani DV. Vascular and biliary variants in the liver: implications for liver surgery. Radiographics. 2008;28:359–78.
11. Furusawa N, Kobayashi A, Yokoyama T, Shimizu A, Motoyama H, Kanai K, Arakura N, Yamada A, Kitou Y, Miyagawa S-I. Biliary tract variations of the left liver with special reference to the left medial sectional bile duct in 500 patients. Am J Surg. 2015;210:351–6.
12. Grimes N, Mark D, McKie L, Scoffield J, Kirk G, Taylor M, Diamond T. Anomalous biliary and vascular anatomy-potential pitfalls during cholecystectomy. Clin Anat. 2017;30:1103–6.
13. Merh R, Saunders M, Jenner D. One duct, two orifices, no names! The anatomy of the biliary cystic duct. Clin Anat. 2018;31:422–3.
14. Schnelldorfer T, Sarr MG, Adams DB. What is the duct of Luschka?–a systematic review. J Gastrointest Surg. 2012;16:656–62.
15. Handra-Luca A, Ben Romdhane HM, Hong S-M. Luschka ducts of the gallbladder in adults: case series report and review of the medical literature. Int J Surg Pathol. 2020;28:482–9.
16. Laurenzi A, Allard M-A, Vibert E. Hepaticocholecystic duct: a pitfall of cholecystectomy. Clin Case Rep. 2019;7:227–8.
17. Crist DW, Gadacz TR. Laparoscopic anatomy of the biliary tree. Surg Clin North Am. 1993;73:785–98.
18. Adams DB. The importance of extrahepatic biliary anatomy in preventing complications at laparoscopic cholecystectomy. Surg Clin North Am. 1993;73:861–71.

Chapter 3
Prevention

Juan Pekolj

The analysis and implementation strategies in preventing BDIs are not a simple task, considering that they are usually generated after a series of decisions made by individuals who are going through heterogeneous and complex scenarios.

Nevertheless, interventions aiming to avoid or mitigate the catastrophic consequences of a single BDI will be fully justified.

When analyzing prevention in BDIs, as if we were discussing any disease, we find it reasonable to stratify it in the classic four levels as follows:

Primary Prevention It is the most important level since it aims to prevent the generation of a BDI.

The primary prevention in BDIs involves "performing the surgery correctly." This is likely achieved by having the regional anatomy ("Critical View of Safety") well-identified, performing safe hemostatic maneuvers, using Intraoperative Cholangiography (IOC), and having a low threshold for deciding to stop the surgery and performing alternative procedures to total cholecystectomy if necessary [1, 2].

Adequate training is essential to primarily prevent a BDI and can be properly performed both in surgery residency and post-residency. There is solid evidence that the "learning curve" for Laparoscopic Cholecystectomy (LC) is hardly reached at the end of the residency. Therefore, we believe is key preparing our trainees to be always cautious and humble [3, 4].

However, it has been seen that the learning curve is not everything. Archer et al. found that training obviously decreased injuries associated with the learning curve, but not those occurring after two hundred LC, what they called " the expert injuries"

J. Pekolj (✉)
General Surgery Service & Liver, Transplant Unit, Buenos Aires, Buenos Aires, Argentina
e-mail: juan.pekolj@hospitalitaliano.org.ar

J. Pekolj et al. (eds.), *Fundamentals of Bile Duct Injuries*,
https://doi.org/10.1007/978-3-031-13383-1_3

[5]. The reasons for these are hard to explain but surely can vary from expert surgeons taking care of more complex cases, to routine cases managed with overconfidence. Bottom line is that a BDI can occur with any degree of expertise [6, 7].

In the same work, surgeons who used IOC recognized 81% of their injuries, while for those who did not use IOC only 45% were able to identify a BDI during the primary procedure [5].

The IOC has an unquestionable role to play in terms of prevention, intraoperative diagnosis, and prevention of complex injuries since identifying the anatomy with more clarity, it is possible to avoid erroneous dissection and injuring more vital structures [8].

Moreover, population-based studies have shown that the rate of BDI was twice higher in populations where IOC is not routinely used [9].

Although injuries may occur after IOC, they are very rare. Almost 30 years after our publication regarding its routine applicability in LC, we believe that the concepts we opportunely expressed are still in force (Fig. 3.1) [10].

Fluorescence cholangiogram represents a promising alternative, although is not currently widely utilized. It consists of using a fluorescent substance (p.e Indocyanine Green) that is injected intravenously and after a few minutes (biliary phase) is excreted through the biliary tract. This, along with a light source, optics and camera head specially adapted and capable of reading the fluorescence, the identification of the bile ducts without prior dissection can be possible, allowing a better interpretation of the anatomy [11].

Alternative procedures such as subtotal or partial cholecystectomy are valid techniques to treat gallbladder pathology in the presence of advanced inflammatory processes with unclear regional anatomy.

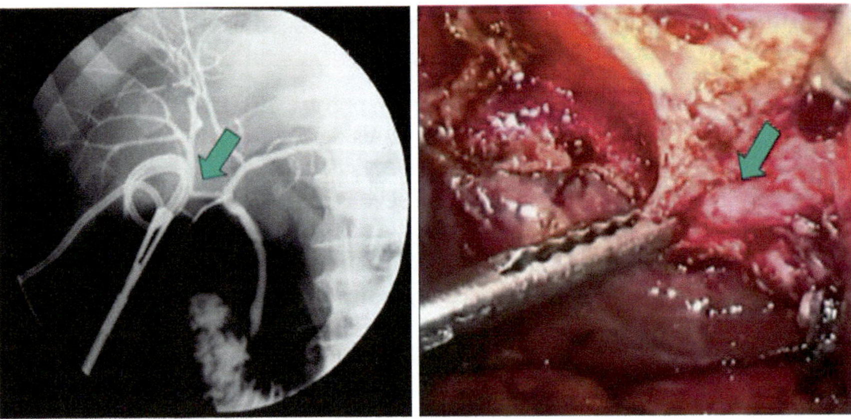

Fig. 3.1 IOC in a patient with previous percutaneous cholecystostomy showing angulation of the right posterior bile duct on the traction of the gallbladder infundibulum. Upon this finding, a partial cholecystectomy was performed leaving a gallbladder cap at the liver bed. The green arrow shows this duct in the IOC and in the laparoscopic view. Without the information facilitated by the IOC, there would have been an injury to the mentioned duct

In the case of conversion to open surgery, it is important to keep in mind that the risk of BDI is high. Targarona et al. showed that this risk was 2.5% in converted LC when the rates in open or laparoscopic surgery were respectively lower (0.5% and 0.8%, respectively, $p < 0.05$) [12]. This higher incidence is explained by the fact that converted patients include cases with hemorrhage, in which the surgeon must act quickly, in a more complex scenario usually characterized by advanced inflammatory processes and a markedly distorted regional anatomy.

Three Main Pillars to Primary Prevent a BDI

1. Having all the necessary equipment in perfect condition including fluoroscopy for IOC.
2. Patient selection must be related to the degree of training.
3. Low threshold for considering alternative techniques to total cholecystectomy if necessary [2].

Technical Recommendations

1. To use 30° optics as it provides depth sensation and better exposure of the cystic and Porta Hepatis simultaneously.
2. The grasping of the vesicular fundus should not be cephalic and medial, but cephalic and lateral (Fig. 3.2a).
3. Traction from the Hartmann's pouch should be made caudally and laterally, to open the area of the cystic pedicle triangle (Fig. 3.2b).
4. Dissection of the cystic duct should be performed at its junction with the infundibulum.

   The CD/CBD junction should not be explored, as this increases the possibility of a BDI. The myth of the long cystic duct syndrome should be set aside. We must remember that a cystic duct that is thick, that is well irrigated, that reaches the pancreas is NOT A CYSTIC DUCT!!! (Fig. 3.3) [13].
5. Prior to the section of any element, the two elements of the cystic pedicle (CA and CD) must be completely identified using blunt maneuvers (Strassberg Critical Safety View) [1].
6. The systematic use of IOC is highly recommended. This is not a panacea, but it allows the identification of anatomical that could predispose to injuries. When an injury occurred, the IOC is not only useful for diagnosis but prevents the progression to a more serious injury. If the surgeon erroneously places the cholangiography catheter in the CBD, assuming that is the CD, although having a correct interpretation of the fluoroscopy findings, it will not continue with the error, and resection of the bile duct will be avoided [14, 9].

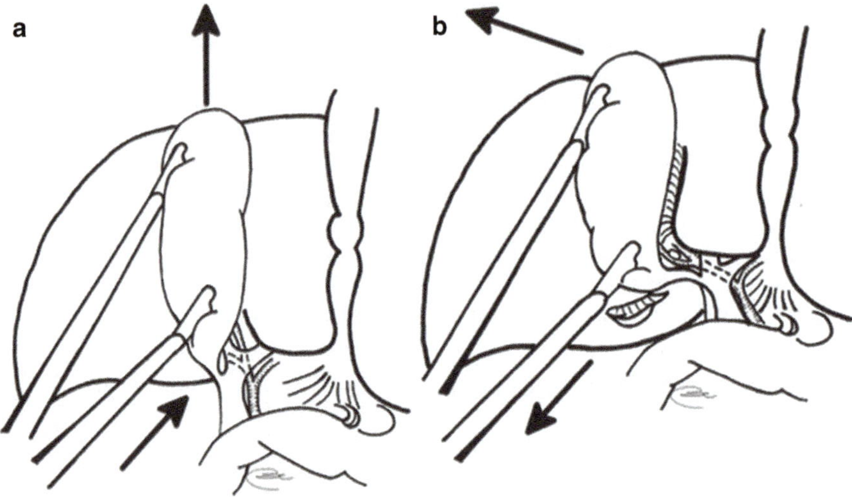

Fig. 3.2 (**a**) Inadequate traction for exposure of the hepato-cystic triangle (**b**) Adequate gallbladder traction for exposure of the hepato-cystic triangle

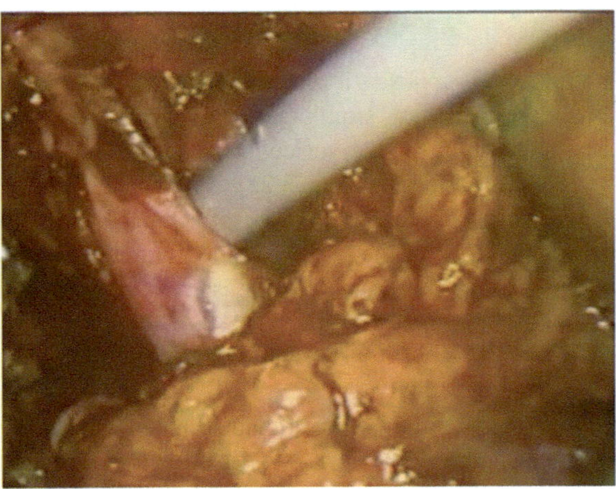

Fig. 3.3 Laparoscopic image of the common bile duct that was interpreted as a cystic duct in a patient with previous gastrectomy and Mirizzi syndrome type II. This erroneous interpretation led to resection of the bile duct, which was solved with hepaticojejunal anastomosis in the same surgery

Secondary Prevention Refers to the early diagnosis of a BDI in order to limit their deleterious effects, extension, and progression. In these situations, intraoperative diagnosis of injuries is key to preventing the progression of unnoticed injuries, which are the most life threatening for patients [15].

In these scenarios the role of IOC is indisputable. It facilitates the diagnosis of BDI and prevents further damage to the porta hepatis structures (Fig. 3.4).

In two publications by our group, we demonstrated that in 80% of BDI the first manifestation of a suspected BDI was abnormal findings in the IOC. In addition,

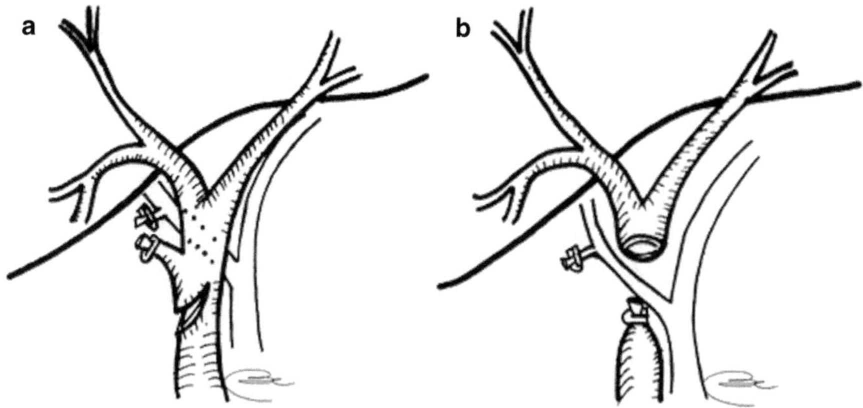

Fig. 3.4 The IOC, by diagnosing anatomical confusion at cannulation, avoids further biliary injury that may lead to bile duct resection with potential associated arterial damage. (**a**) Minor BDI after miscannulation for IOC. The injury no progress due to the intraoperative diagnosis, (**b**) Major BDI by misinterpretation of the anatomy and no use of IOC

when the IOC was motivated by the evidence of a bile leak, the diagnosis of the precise situation causing the leak was cleared out in 90% of cases [9].

Intraoperative diagnosis equals prompt repair. The latter performed by trained surgeons ensure long-term effectiveness greater than 90%.

In combination, these factors determine a better postoperative course, with less morbidity and sequelae, and with less alteration of the quality of life and, extremely important, risk of mortality [16].

It is worth mentioning that these factors are related to a lower litigation rate, as has been published in numerous international series.

Figure 3.5 summarizes the purposes of secondary prevention and its benefits.

Tertiary Prevention Refers to installing appropriate and opportune-directed therapies to avoid complications and sequelae away from repair procedures. As it is popularly said, "to prevent the remedy from being worse than the disease."

The surgeon who diagnoses a BDI intraoperatively must answer himself/herself these difficult questions:

1. Am I properly equipped to obtain an adequate IOC?
2. Do I feel comfortable performing a primary repair or a biliodigestive anastomosis to the proximal biliary tree with a normal caliber, thin-walled bile duct?
3. Would it be better managed by concluding the surgery at that point, placing abdominal drains, and referring the patient to a tertiary center upon discussion of the situation with the patient and their family?

This is extremely important as it determines the outcome of these patients. In a review of a national survey in the USA by Archer et al., it was found that only

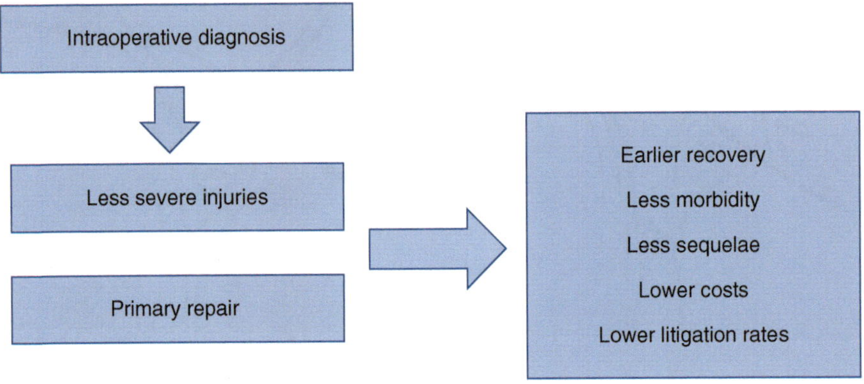

Fig. 3.5 Objectives and advantages of secondary prevention in BDIs

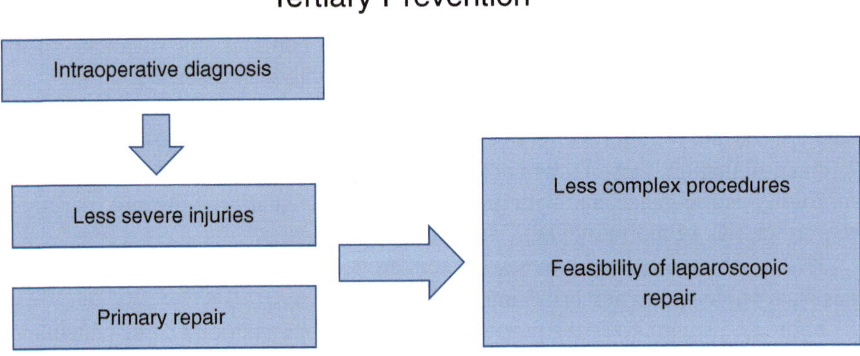

Fig. 3.6 Objectives and advantages of tertiary prevention in BDIs

14.7% of the injuries were referred to referral centers [5]. Figure 3.6 summarizes the purposes and advantages of tertiary prevention in BDI.

Quaternary Prevention This is a more contemporary concept than the aforementioned three and refers to the set of activities that are carried out to prevent, reduce or mitigate the harm caused by their exposure to healthcare. In the case of BDIs, quaternary prevention consists of avoiding the patient's exposure to the risk of suffering a BDI. Discussing the indications for LC more specifically: Why it should be indicated in cases of asymptomatic lithiasis? or, Why it should be indicated in gallbladder polyps below the criteria for malignization? [17].

References

1. Strasberg SM. Avoidance of biliary injury during laparoscopic cholecystectomy. J Hepato-Biliary-Pancreat Surg. 2002;9:543–7.
2. van de Graaf FW, Zaïmi I, Stassen LPS, Lange JF. Safe laparoscopic cholecystectomy: a systematic review of bile duct injury prevention. Int J Surg. 2018;60:164–72.
3. Martin RF, Rossi RL. Bile duct injuries: Spectrum, mechanisms of injury, and their prevention. Surg Clin N Am. 1994;74:781–803.
4. Calvete J, Sabater L, Camps B, Verdú A, Gomez-Portilla A, Martín J, Torrico MA, Flor B, Cassinello N, Lledó S. Bile duct injury during laparoscopic cholecystectomy: myth or reality of the learning curve? Surg Endosc. 2000;14:608–11.
5. Archer SB, Brown DW, Smith CD, Branum GD, Hunter JG. Bile duct injury during laparoscopic cholecystectomy: results of a national survey. Ann Surg. 2001;234(549–58):discussion 558–9.
6. McKinley SK, Brunt LM, Schwaitzberg SD. Prevention of bile duct injury: the case for incorporating educational theories of expertise. Surg Endosc. 2014;28:3385–91.
7. Dekker SWA, Hugh TB. Laparoscopic bile duct injury: understanding the psychology and heuristics of the error. ANZ J Surg. 2008;78:1109–14.
8. Buddingh KT, Nieuwenhuijs VB, van Buuren L, Hulscher JBF, de Jong JS, van Dam GM. Intraoperative assessment of biliary anatomy for prevention of bile duct injury: a review of current and future patient safety interventions. Surg Endosc. 2011;25:2449–61.
9. Alvarez FA, de Santibañes M, Palavecino M, Sánchez Clariá R, Mazza O, Arbues G, de Santibañes E, Pekolj J. Impact of routine intraoperative cholangiography during laparoscopic cholecystectomy on bile duct injury. Br J Surg. 2014;101:677–84.
10. Pekolj J, Santibáñes E de, Sívori JA, Ciardullo MA, Campi O, Mazzaro E (1993) La colangiografía transcística durante la colecistectomía laparoscópica. Rev Argent Cir 5–11.
11. Ankersmit M, van Dam DA, van Rijswijk A-S, van den Heuvel B, Tuynman JB, Meijerink WJHJ. Fluorescent imaging with Indocyanine green during laparoscopic cholecystectomy in patients at increased risk of bile duct injury. Surg Innov. 2017;24:245–52.
12. Targarona EM, Marco C, Balagué C, Rodriguez J, Cugat E, Hoyuela C, Veloso E, Trias M. How, when, and why bile duct injury occurs. A comparison between open and laparoscopic cholecystectomy. Surg Endosc. 1998;12:322–6.
13. Gupta V, Jain G. Safe laparoscopic cholecystectomy: adoption of universal culture of safety in cholecystectomy. World J Gastrointest Surg. 2019;11:62–84.
14. Michael Brunt L, Deziel DJ, Telem DA, et al. Safe cholecystectomy multi-society practice guideline and state-of-the-art consensus conference on prevention of bile duct injury during cholecystectomy. Surg Endosc. 2020;34:2827–55.
15. Rystedt JML, Montgomery AK. Quality-of-life after bile duct injury: intraoperative detection is crucial. A National Case-Control Study HPB. 2016;18:1010–6.
16. Pekolj J, Alvarez FA, Palavecino M, Sánchez Clariá R, Mazza O, de Santibañes E. Intraoperative management and repair of bile duct injuries sustained during 10,123 laparoscopic cholecystectomies in a high-volume referral center. J Am Coll Surg. 2013;216:894–901.
17. Zha Y, Chen X-R, Luo D, Jin Y. The prevention of major bile duct injures in laparoscopic cholecystectomy: the experience with 13,000 patients in a single center. Surg Laparosc Endosc Percutan Tech. 2010;20:378–83.

Chapter 4
Essential Aspects BDI Management

Oscar Mazza and Marcos Zandomeni

Most BDIs are complex for nonspecialist surgeons and can become more complex when they are treated inappropriately. They can lead to serious complications such as peritonitis, sepsis, and multi-organ failure in the early stages; or cholangitis, secondary biliary cirrhosis (SBC) that would require a repeated ERCPs (Endoscopic Retrograde Cholangiopancreatography), percutaneous transhepatic cholangiogram and percutaneous biliary drainage (PTC/PBD), liver resections or more rare liver transplantation (LT) down the road [1].

Although there is certainly extensive literature regarding BDIs, there is no clear standardization about the best approach in individual cases. And this is just because it depends on multiple variables that must be considered:

- The time and manner of diagnosis.
- The mechanism and type of injury.
- The local characteristics.
- The systemic impact on the patient.
- The training and psychological impact of the BDI on the responsible surgeon (Fig. 4.1).

We have therefore determined the Levels of Prevention that must be considered to successfully prevent, treat and manage the complications of BDI (Fig. 4.2).

Although this organization has been described in Chap. 3, we will use a similar structure but with a special focus on the basic aspects of BDI management.

O. Mazza (✉)
HPB Surgery, General Surgery Service, Hospital Italiano de Buenos Aires, Buenos Aires, Argentina
e-mail: oscar.mazza@hospitalitaliano.org.ar

M. Zandomeni
General and HPB Surgery, Hospital Durand, Buenos Aires, Argentina

J. Pekolj et al. (eds.), *Fundamentals of Bile Duct Injuries*, https://doi.org/10.1007/978-3-031-13383-1_4

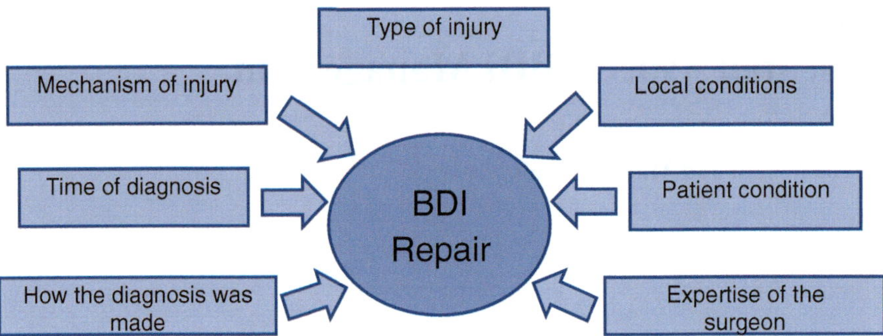

Fig. 4.1 Different factors that have a direct impact on the repair of a bile duct injuries

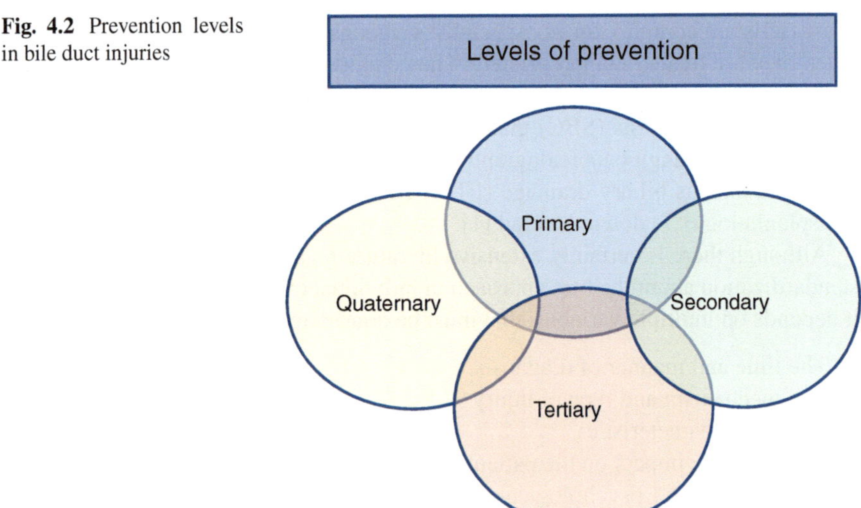

Fig. 4.2 Prevention levels in bile duct injuries

Primary Prevention

Primary prevention consists of avoiding a BDI from the outset and, limiting its progression and or extension once it occurred (Fig. 4.3). A correct interpretation of the normal anatomy and understanding of the most frequent variations is key for this instance [2].

Multiple surgical techniques have been described for the prevention of a BDI: the Infundibular technique; Strasberg's critical view; exposure of the common bile duct (CBD), correct traction of the gallbladder infundibulum; intraoperative cholangiography (IOC), etc. [3]. Although no technique is infallible, the trained surgeon should be acquainted with them in case the situation demands the application of any [4].

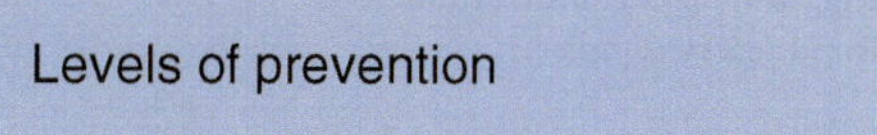

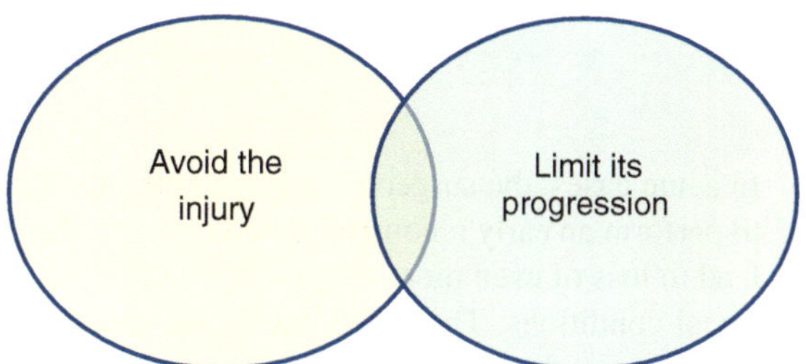

Fig. 4.3 Primary prevention in bile duct injuries

We consider the routine IOC one of our best allies, as it permits a thorough mapping of the biliary tree; and in the case of an inadverted BDI, it enables us to diagnose them at the time of the primary surgery, and ultimately can prevent its progression in 90% of the cases [5].

In a literature review, Buddingh et al. established that in more than 900 cholecystectomies the incidence of major BDI (Strasberg E) in patients who underwent selective IOC was 1.9%, whereas when systematic IOC was performed it was 0%. This is because once BDI was detected, total section, resection, or thermal injury of the bile duct could be avoided [6].

Secondary Prevention

Secondary prevention consists of early diagnosis and correct repair of the BDI. Each unsuccessful attempt is associated with shortening the non-injured bile duct and may even result in amputation of the right and left hepatic ducts that were not initially involved. Successive episodes of cholangitis can compromise both the overall condition (nutrition, sepsis) of the patient and predispose to progressive fibrosis of the liver. Therefore, these factors increase the overall failure rate of any intervention [7].

It is important to consider certain conditions for early repair of a BDI (Fig. 4.4):

- Mechanism of Injury: If the *injury* is ischemic by nature, such as those produced by a thermal instrument, early repair is likely to be unsuccessful. The reason is that an ischemic BDI usually progresses over time and the real damaged area becomes larger. Therefore, any repair in this location is likely to be compromised, leading to necrosis and subsequent dehiscence of the eventual reconstruction/anastomosis [8].

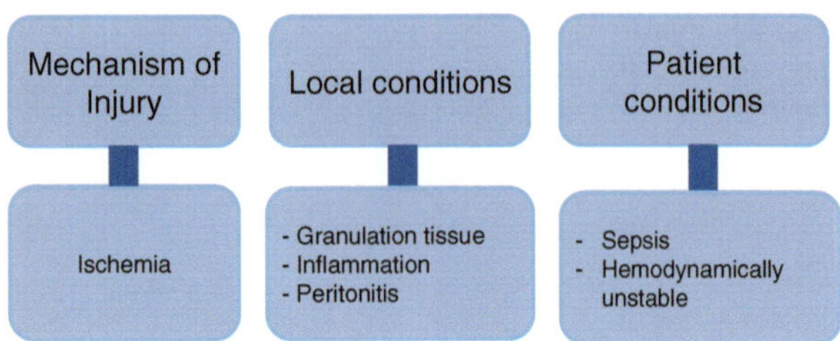

Fig. 4.4 Contraindications for an early repair

- In acute cases, the surgeon can be tempted to refresh the edges of the bile ducts to perform an early reconstruction. However, this is extremely imprecise and can lead to loss of even more ductal length [9].
- Local conditions: The condition of the abdominal cavity at the moment of the repair can undoubtedly play a role in the ultimate outcome. Attempting a repair in granulation tissue, with local inflammation, friable tissues, or in the context of biliary peritonitis determines a poor-quality anastomosis and an increased incidence of failure.
- Patient condition: In the case of septic patients with hemodynamic instability, all the therapies should be directed toward the cause of their current condition (cholangitis, biliary peritonitis, bacteremia). Considering doing a complex surgery such as bile duct repair is absolutely contraindicated [10].

As mentioned above, early and precise diagnosis is achieved most of the time through the use of IOC. In a manuscript published by our group, we observed that out of 11,423 Laparoscopic Cholecystectomies (LC) we presented 20 BDI; 90% were detected intraoperatively which allowed a repair during the same procedure [11, 12].

If the diagnosis is made post-surgery, an early or late repair can be performed, assessing each case individually.

"Early repair" is defined as that performed within the first 7 postoperative days after LC. "Late repair" is that BDI repair performed beyond 6–8 weeks. However, reconstructive procedures in the time window in between these (7 days to 6 weeks postoperatively) should be precluded, as there is clear data supporting the worst time to attempt a repair given the postoperative locoregional condition [13].

We then move on to the second point of secondary prevention, the correct repair of the bile duct. Perhaps one of the most difficult and important decisions in BDI management is selecting appropriately the right moment for the repair. This will vary according to the time of diagnosis: *intraoperative or postoperative*.

Intraoperative Diagnosis

In centers where selective IOC was performed, only 15–30% of biliary lesions are identified intraoperatively. The BDI is identified by evidence of an obvious bile leak or by an abnormal IOC.

The surgeon should carefully consider their experience and skill to repair it. Our recommendation is that a reasonable course of action in the first instance would be to call in a more experienced surgeon or, otherwise, a surgeon with the same experience, but without the stress of having caused a BDI. If help is not available, but with the necessary experience, the surgeon may attempt to handle the case themself.

However, when a BDI is identified and the acting surgeon is unable to repair it, the subphrenic and subhepatic spaces should be adequately drained and referred to a center with hepatobiliary specialists [14]. The well-known phrase *"I drain, and I'm gone!"* was popularized by Dr. Pekolj in numerous lectures.

Postoperative Diagnosis

Initially, the clinical manifestations of DBI must be managed aggressively. In case of bile leak, biloma (infected or not), or choleperitoneum, it will require percutaneous or laparoscopic drainage of the affected spaces [15, 16].

If the clinical manifestation involves cholestasis or cholangitis, it can be managed with conservative measures, antibiotics, or eventually draining the bile duct through a PTC/PBD or ERCP [17].

The next course of action is to determine the type of injury we are dealing with. For this, Magnetic Resonance Cholangiopancreatography (MRCP) is an extremely useful noninvasive method or if there is a biliary drain in place, by a cholangiogram with radiopaque dye injection through the drain or ERCP. Depending on the mechanism of injury, it may also be appropriate to perform a Computed Tomography (CT) scan with angiography to rule out any associated vascular injury, in particular, of the right hepatic artery (RHA) [17, 18].

Early Repair

In case of a partial or total section without thermal injury, primary suture or end-to-end anastomosis may be performed with or without biliary drainage. In case of bile duct resection or thermal injury, an inexperienced surgeon will obtain better results by performing correct drainage of the cavity (right subphrenic and subhepatic spaces) and referring the patient. An experienced surgeon in this scenario will be able to perform a resection of the margins and eventually hepaticojejunostomy if the locoregional conditions are favorable [19].

In general terms, a correct exposure of the damaged area is suggested, avoiding excessive dissection of the porta hepatis, in order to avoid irreversible injuries. The biliary duct should be free of retractions or thermal lesions. In all cases, we suggest performing IOC for a correct delimitation of the extent of the lesion. The integrity of the vascular structures, in particular, the RHA and hepatic artery (HA) and the PV, should be confirmed. If the situation is deemed favorable, a hepaticojejunostomy under magnification with a slowly resorbing suture can be performed [20, 21].

Late Repair

It is advisable to defer the repair (beyond 6–8 weeks) in case of late presentation of the injury, previous failed attempts to repair it, the presence of biliary peritonitis, clinical instability, or in the context of a severe thermal injury [22].

When we are dealing with an unsuccessful BDI repair, the patient must undergo an exhaustive study to prevent future failures. In these cases, the workup must include a CT scan with angiography to assess the indemnity of the RHA, as its associated injury is directly associated with restenosis of a BDI repair [23].

In a study examining autopsies of cholecystectomised patients, 7% were found to have some type of vascular injury. However, most of the time the HA ligation can be well tolerated when the PV flow is preserved, along with continuity of collateral circulation via the hilar plexus. On the contrary, the total or partial HA disruption can lead to ischemic cholangiopathy or even acute hepatic infarction, which will depend on the individual collateralization of the patient, atherosclerosis, etc. [24].

Tertiary Prevention

Tertiary prevention consists of moderating the sequelae of a BDI, improving the patient's quality of life, and preventing the development of secondary biliary cirrhosis (SBC) (Fig. 4.5).

In progressive cases with recurrent cholangitis due to varying degrees of biliary stenosis, the first step is to optimize the biliary outflow by PBD. If there is continuity of the biliary duct, balloon dilatation of the stenosis is attempted in our center with a 90% success rate a year [25]; if this is unsuccessful, the patient must be assessed in an experienced center, where hepaticojejunal or cholangiojejunal anastomosis may be considered [26].

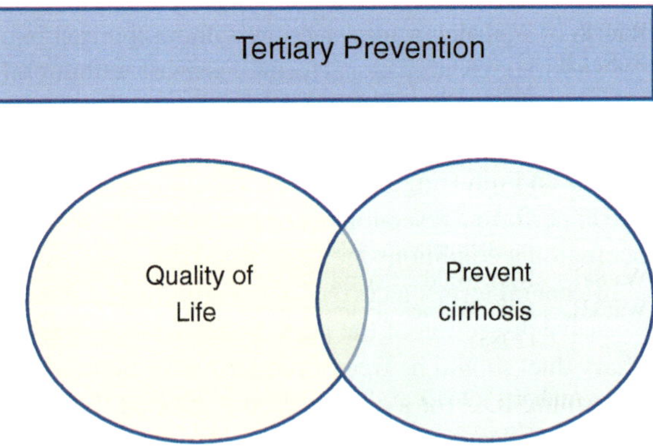

Fig. 4.5 Tertiary prevention in bile duct injuries

Nevertheless, ***liver resection*** could also be considered in cases with:

- Second-order biliary duct stenosis.
- Biliary confluence stenosis with ipsilateral vascular injury.
- A simultaneous ipsilateral arterial and portal injury extended intrahepatic stenosis without continuity with the biliary duct.
- Lobar atrophy with infected hepatic necrosis and ipsilateral intrahepatic lithiasis.

Multiple failed repair attempts or inappropriate treatment of chronic cholestasis and multiple infections can ultimately create fertile soil for SBC, in general, several years after the BDI [27].

In a historical series of BDI repairs, the incidence of biliary hypertension and SBC has been 8%.

The presence of cirrhosis during attempted biliary duct repair is considered an ominous sign and an outstanding risk factor in increased mortality among different series. When there is a suspicion of liver fibrosis the patient should be referred to a specialized center with LT capacity [28].

In patients with complex BDI and concomitant portal hypertension, although preserved biliary-enteric continuity, interventional radiology approaches play a crucial role in their management. If there is no continuity and the patient has contraindications to LT, the biliary duct is drained by percutaneous drainage, and portal hypertension is treated medically, with TIPS or less likely mesocaval shunt [29].

Most of the histological changes performed in the early stages of obstruction are usually reversible if they are treated on time. The following are all decompensating features of chronic and irreversible liver disease and therefore, the need for LT: refractory ascites, gastrointestinal hemorrhage from esophageal varices, encephalopathy, recurrent cholangitis, progressive jaundice, uncontrollable pruritus, and poor quality of life [30, 31].

Quaternary Prevention

In recent years, this concept of quaternary prevention became in vogue. According to its definition, *"an action taken to identify patients at risk of hyper-medicalization, to protect them from further medical invasion and to suggest ethically acceptable procedures."*

How can this concept be applied to BDIs?

The answer seems simple, but perhaps difficult to generalize. Multiple reports following the development of LC have shown that the mini-invasive approach led to an increase in the number of practices performed worldwide. The origin of this surge was not only due to the fact that patients were more likely to choose laparoscopic treatment because of less parietal aggression and fewer aesthetic defects compared to the open approach, but also due to a subjective appreciation of less surgical aggression by the surgeon himself.

This led to a less severe indication for surgical treatment. Contrary to original expectations, most reports of large surgical experiences have demonstrated a sustained increase in the incidence of BDI with the laparoscopic approach. In some reports, the incidence of these injuries was up to ten times higher than in the open era.

Far from criticizing MIS surgery, the point is to emphasize the correct indications for surgery, recognizing that even in the easiest elective cholecystectomies there is a real possibility of BDI and their deemed consequences. Consequently, the risk must be justified and the patient adequately selected.

The expertise of the surgeon must be considered as well. An elderly patient with asymptomatic lithiasis who is taken to the operating room, or an obese patient with subacute cholecystitis operated on by an undertrained surgeon may be illustrative of an act of prevention before taking the patient to a procedure that is not properly indicated.

Conclusions

BDI casts a pall of uncertainty over a patient's quality of life and prognosis. Prevention of this iatrogenic disease is based on making the right decision at the right time. Detailed knowledge of the anatomy and its variants as well as the systematic performance of IOC are initial elements that help to reduce not only the incidence of lesions but also the generation of more serious and complex ones.

Once the injury has been produced, the surgeon must be able to evaluate the opportunity and most appropriate technique for repair, either in the same surgical act or by deferring the repair to another time or even another trained surgeon. The goal is not to increase the damage with unsuccessful attempts at repair.

The prevention of long-term sequelae involves a strict follow-up of the patient in order to detect possible liver complications due to stenosis or dysfunction of the anastomosis that may lead to chronic cholestasis with possible evolution to fibrosis or cirrhosis.

Finally, the first prevention is to perform the right surgery on the right patient with the right surgical indication.

References

1. van de Graaf FW, Zaïmi I, Stassen LPS, Lange JF. Safe laparoscopic cholecystectomy: a systematic review of bile duct injury prevention. Int J Surg. 2018;60:164–72.
2. Dumot JA. Injury of the aberrant bile duct: beware of what you don't see. Gastrointest Endosc. 2020;91:593–4.
3. Wysocki AP. Population-based studies should not be used to justify a policy of routine cholangiography to prevent major bile duct injury during laparoscopic cholecystectomy. World J Surg. 2017;41:82–9.

4. Michael Brunt L, Deziel DJ, Telem DA, et al. Safe cholecystectomy multi-society practice guideline and state-of-the-art consensus conference on prevention of bile duct injury during cholecystectomy. Surg Endosc. 2020;34:2827–55.
5. Alvarez FA, de Santibañes M, Palavecino M, Sánchez Clariá R, Mazza O, Arbues G, de Santibañes E, Pekolj J. Impact of routine intraoperative cholangiography during laparoscopic cholecystectomy on bile duct injury. Br J Surg. 2014;101:677–84.
6. Buddingh KT, Nieuwenhuijs VB, van Buuren L, Hulscher JBF, de Jong JS, van Dam GM. Intraoperative assessment of biliary anatomy for prevention of bile duct injury: a review of current and future patient safety interventions. Surg Endosc. 2011;25:2449–61.
7. Nordin A, Halme L, Mäkisalo H, Isoniemi H, Höckerstedt K. Management and outcome of major bile duct injuries after laparoscopic cholecystectomy: from therapeutic endoscopy to liver transplantation. Liver Transpl. 2002;8:1036–43.
8. Nechay T, Sazhin A, Titkova S, Anurov M, Tyagunov A, Sheptunov S, Yakhutlov U, Nakhushev R, Sannikov A. Thermal processes in bile ducts during laparoscopic cholecystectomy with monopolar instruments. experimental study using real-time intraluminal and surface thermography. Surg Innov. 2021;28:525–35.
9. Mercado MA, Chan C, Orozco H, Tielve M, Hinojosa CA. Acute bile duct injury. The need for a high repair. Surg Endosc. 2003;17:1351–5.
10. de'Angelis N, Catena F, Memeo R, et al. 2020 WSES guidelines for the detection and management of bile duct injury during cholecystectomy. World J Emerg Surg. 2021;16:30.
11. Christou N, Roux-David A, Naumann DN, et al. Bile duct injury during cholecystectomy: necessity to learn how to do and interpret intraoperative cholangiography. Front Med. 2021;8:637987.
12. Pekolj J, Alvarez FA, Palavecino M, Sánchez Clariá R, Mazza O, de Santibañes E. Intraoperative management and repair of bile duct injuries sustained during 10,123 laparoscopic cholecystectomies in a high-volume referral center. J Am Coll Surg. 2013;216:894–901.
13. Felekouras E, Petrou A, Neofytou K, Moris D, Dimitrokallis N, Bramis K, Griniatsos J, Pikoulis E, Diamantis T. Early or delayed intervention for bile duct injuries following laparoscopic cholecystectomy? A dilemma looking for an answer. Gastroenterol Res Pract. 2015;2015:104235.
14. Martinez-Lopez S, Upasani V, Pandanaboyana S, Attia M, Toogood G, Lodge P, Hidalgo E. Delayed referral to specialist centre increases morbidity in patients with bile duct injury (BDI) after laparoscopic cholecystectomy (LC). Int J Surg. 2017;44:82–6.
15. Gupta V, Jayaraman S. Role for laparoscopy in the management of bile duct injuries. Can J Surg. 2017;60:300–4.
16. Pekolj J, Drago J. Controversies in iatrogenic bile duct injuries. Role of video-assisted laparoscopy in the management of iatrogenic bile duct injuries. Cir Esp. 2020;98:61–3.
17. Pawa S, Al-Kawas FH. ERCP in the management of biliary complications after cholecystectomy. Curr Gastroenterol Rep. 2009;11:160–6.
18. Ragozzino A, De Ritis R, Mosca A, Iaccarino V, Imbriaco M. Value of MR cholangiography in patients with iatrogenic bile duct injury after cholecystectomy. Am J Roentgenol. 2004;183:1567–72.
19. de Santibáñes E, Ardiles V, Pekolj J. Complex bile duct injuries: management. HPB. 2008;10:4–12.
20. Roncati L, Manenti A, Zizzo M, Manco G, Farinetti A. Complex bile duct injury: when to repair. Surgery. 2019;165:486–96.
21. Stewart L, Way LW. Laparoscopic bile duct injuries: timing of surgical repair does not influence success rate. A multivariate analysis of factors influencing surgical outcomes. HPB. 2009;11:516–22.
22. Wang X, Yu W-L, Fu X-H, Zhu B, Zhao T, Zhang Y-J. Early versus delayed surgical repair and referral for patients with bile duct injury: a systematic review and meta-analysis. Ann Surg. 2020;271:449–59.
23. Booij KAC, Coelen RJ, de Reuver PR, Besselink MG, van Delden OM, Rauws EA, Busch OR, van Gulik TM, Gouma DJ. Long-term follow-up and risk factors for strictures after hepaticoje-

junostomy for bile duct injury: an analysis of surgical and percutaneous treatment in a tertiary center. Surgery. 2018;163:1121–7.

24. A European-African HepatoPancreatoBiliary Association (E-AHPBA) Research Collaborative Study management group, Other members of the European-African HepatoPancreatoBiliary Association Research Collaborative. Post cholecystectomy bile duct injury: early, intermediate or late repair with hepaticojejunostomy—an E-AHPBA multi-center study. HPB. 2019;21:1641–7.
25. Czerwonko ME, Huespe P, Mazza O, de Santibanes M, Sanchez-Claria R, Pekolj J, Ciardullo M, de Santibanes E, Hyon SH. Percutaneous biliary balloon dilation: impact of an institutional three-session protocol on patients with benign anastomotic strictures of hepatojejunostomy. Dig Surg. 2018;35:397–405.
26. Martínez-Mier G, Moreno-Ley PI, Mendez-Rico D. Factors associated with patency loss and actuarial patency rate following post-cholecystectomy bile duct injury repair: long-term follow-up. Langenbecks Arch Surg. 2020;405:999–1006.
27. Khadra H, Johnson H, Crowther J, McClaren P, Darden M, Parker G, Buell JF. Bile duct injury repairs: progressive outcomes in a tertiary referral center. Surgery. 2019;166:698–702.
28. El Nakeeb A, Sultan A, Ezzat H, Attia M, Abd ElWahab M, Kayed T, Hassanen A, AlMalki A, Alqarni A, Mohammed MM. Impact of referral pattern and timing of repair on surgical outcome after reconstruction of post-cholecystectomy bile duct injury: a multicenter study. Hepatobiliary Pancreat Dis Int. 2021;20:53–60.
29. Negi SS, Sakhuja P, Malhotra V, Chaudhary A. Factors predicting advanced hepatic fibrosis in patients with postcholecystectomy bile duct strictures. Arch Surg. 2004;139:299–303.
30. Schreuder AM, Busch OR, Besselink MG, Ignatavicius P, Gulbinas A, Barauskas G, Gouma DJ, van Gulik TM. Long-term impact of iatrogenic bile duct injury. Dig Surg. 2020;37:10–21.
31. Moore DE, Feurer ID, Holzman MD, Wudel LJ, Strickland C, Gorden DL, Chari R, Wright JK, Pinson CW. Long-term detrimental effect of bile duct injury on health-related quality of life. Arch Surg. 2004;139:476–81; discussion 481–2.

Chapter 5
Physiopathology of BDI

Martin Palavecino

Introduction

Since the introduction of LC at the end of the 1980s, the increased incidence and complexity of BDI are undeniable [1, 2].

Since then, many efforts have been directed toward a better understanding of the diverse and usually interacting *mechanisms* of injury, in order to try to prevent or eventually, eliminate them.

The term *"Mechanism"* (from Latin "mechanisma") is defined through *objects interacting within a complex structure to produce an effect,* whereas *"Injury"* (from Latin laesión) *denotes an abnormal change in a part of the organism produced by external or internal damage.*

The purpose of this chapter is to describe and analyze the current main mechanisms that favor or predispose to BDIs.

Physiopathology of BDIs

A BDI is one of the most serious complications of LC. It is only exceeded in severity by large vessel injuries and unnoticed hollow viscus injuries [3]. However, by prevalence, a BDI is the leading cause of mortality associated with the laparoscopic management of biliary diseases. Their incidence ranges from 0.3 to 0.5% in the laparoscopic approach, while in the conventional approach, the rate is slightly lower at 0.2–0.3% [4].

M. Palavecino (✉)
HPB Surgery, General Surgery Service, Hospital Italiano de San Justo, San Justo, Argentina
e-mail: martin.palavecino@hospitalitaliano.org.ar

J. Pekolj et al. (eds.), *Fundamentals of Bile Duct Injuries*,
https://doi.org/10.1007/978-3-031-13383-1_5

Why Does a Bile Duct Injury Occur?

Medical error is the third leading cause of death in the United States. As with other types of errors, they occur because of the failure of various control mechanisms, known as the "Swiss cheese theory." In a process expecting a certain outcome (in this case the injury-free dissection of Calot's triangle), several control mechanisms have to be carried out in order to attain that expected outcome [5].

However, each control mechanism has weaknesses, and if every single weak point converges within the same process, a consequent failure of the process (BDI) is likely to occur.

The possible catalysts for a BDI depend on, overall, *three subclasses of factors:*

Patient Dependent

Obesity and local modifications associated with acute cholecystitis (AC) or chronic (scleroatrophic gallbladder or Mirizzi syndrome) inflammatory processes are patient-dependent variables that increase the technical complexity of the surgical procedure [6]. It is well documented in the published literature that patients with AC in progress had twice the risk of suffering a BDI compared with patients without it [7].

There is a correlation between the severity classification of AC and the risk of injury. While a mild AC (Tokyo Grade I) does not increase the overall risk of BDI (OR 0.96 95% CI 0.41–2.25), a moderate AC (Tokyo Grade II) increases the risk more than twofold (OR 2.41 95% CI 1.21–4.80). Moreover, a severe AC (Tokyo grade III) has a significant, eightfold increase in the risk of producing a BDI (OR 8.43 95% CI 0.97–72.9). The intention to use IOC reduces the risk of BDI to 52% (OR 0.48, 95% CI 0.29–0.81) [8].

Morbid obesity [2.8 (2.1–4.3); $p = 0.03$] and Age > 65 [1.5 (1.05–2.1); $p = 0.01$] in patients undergoing LC are other significant patient-related factors reported as independent predictors for BDI in multivariate analysis including 1015 patients who suffered a BDI [9].

Institution-Dependent Factors

The accessibility to abdominal MRCP or even dynamic fluoroscopy to perform IOC for those patients that present with abnormal liver function tests (LFTs) represents a great source of preoperative and or intraoperative information that could contribute to preventing a BDI [10].

In fact, MRCP can demonstrate with more than 96% reliability, the preoperative anatomy in the presence of dilated bile ducts, and with more than 90% sensitivity in detecting anatomical variants in cases of non-dilated ducts. Thanks to its high sensitivity (more than 90%) in detecting even also small stones, these findings can guide the strategy of choledochal lithiasis with gallbladder in situ. Nevertheless, it is expensive, time consuming, and not widely available [11, 12].

Dynamic fluoroscopy is easier to get, but its routine application is still widely discussed. Those in favor of its systematic use argue that it allows clear anatomical mapping and avoids serious BDIs. On the other hand, surgeons that advocate for its selective use, argue that it increases operative time and costs, exposes the patient to radiation, and does not seem to prevent minor injuries [13].

However, if IOC is applied only selectively, it may not be used in case of anatomical doubts, due to lack of experience or omission. Correspondingly, the non-routine use of IOC hinders the learning curve for performing and interpreting it when needed during a complex case [14].

Another alternative to identify anatomical variants is fluorescence cholangiography involving the injection of Indocyanine Green (which is selectively eliminated by biliary secretion). It requires a special polarized light source to highlight its presence in the bile. It is a highly promising and cost-effective method that has been documented with good results (90–100% identification of CD, and its junction with the CBD) [15].

Surgeon-Related Factors

The skill and experience of the surgeon and their confidence in dealing with both challenging cases and complications of the surgery (hemorrhage due to vascular damage, injury to neighboring organs, etc.) are obvious risk factors associated with complications and should never be underestimated [16]. However, the attitude of the surgeon toward challenging or overwhelming situations play an important role in generating BDI as well. For example, persist laparoscopically in a difficult case with inadequately recognized anatomy [17, 18].

In both cases, recognizing that surgeon-related factors could play a role in the genesis of a BDI is the first step. If that is the case, it should be shameless to request assistance from a more experienced surgeon and, if this is not possible, place drains and refer the patient to a high-volume center for HPB surgery to prevent further damage is recommended [19, 20].

Types and Mechanisms of Injury

Two types of injury are described separately although can occur at the same time:

Vascular Injury

A vascular injury causes hemorrhage that may be originated in the hepatic parenchyma, in the gallbladder, in the CA, in the normal or aberrant RHA (or Right Posterior Artery in Rouvière's sulcus). More rarely, bleeding from portal structures may occur (portal branches may be reached in segments IV and V through the gallbladder plate) [21].

Injuries to the Middle Hepatic Vein (MHV) at the level of the gallbladder fossa are also very rare [22].

Independently of the source of bleeding, it may not be significant or interfere with the operative area and the surgeon decides to continue with the dissection.

It is worth mentioning that occult bleeding might also occur and only be noticed when it reaches Morrison's space, as this space can accommodate between 50 and 200 cc of blood and still remain unobserved.

On the other side, bleeding can be severe and prevent the surgeon from proceeding with the normal course of the surgery. In this scenario, there is usually a combination of drawbacks: Illumination decrease because of the bleeding itself, frequent suctioning is required, pneumoperitoneum is reduced, the aspirator is clogged, drying is not sufficient, frequent flushing is required, the surgeon feels that the situation is delaying resolution and becomes anxious and angry at the same time. As a consequence, this situation may lead to further bleeding, biliary or intestinal injury, or major damage to the porta hepatis. *Hemorrhage is the most frequent cause of conversion* [23–25].

There are also predisposing factors for bleeding. For instance, inflammatory processes, naturally due to congestion and neovascularization, increase the areas of hemorrhage. Fibrotic, retractile processes not only enclose and hide the vessels but also displace them from their natural disposition [26].

Portal hypertension and acute pancreatitis also contribute to bleeding. The hepatomegaly causes the parenchyma to become friable and the usual separation maneuvers easily injure it.

In minor bleedings, the first step is to perform transient hemostasis. If the bleeding is mild, compression with a regular sponge or Rey-Tec for 2–3 min should suffice.

If a major vascular structure is affected and or the bleeding is beyond the surgeons' control, an appropriate response consists of compressing and simultaneously performing a laparotomy for definitive resolution [27].

Ultimate hemostasis will only be intended after accurate identification of the bleeding source and its correct repair. Otherwise, it would set the field for a BDI.

Therefore, more experienced surgeons or surgeons who are not emotionally involved in the situation should be consulted whenever possible to ensure the situation is properly controlled.

Biliary Injury

The morbidity and mortality of a BDI dramatically rise when it is associated with vascular injury, thermal injury, and/or resection of the CBD.

Although predisposing conditions are not always present, the majority are related to challenging cases.

Injuries are often associated with:

- Misinterpretation of the regional anatomy: when the structures are misread is when a BDI almost certainly occurs [28].
- Hence, the importance of IOC to be certain of what we are dividing is the CD and not anything else like the CBD. "Strasberg's Critical View of Safety" concept is represented by the fact that only two structures (cystic artery and cystic duct) must be clearly attached to the gallbladder Fig. 5.1. If this is misinterpreted, a small lateral section is performed with cautery scissors with the purpose of performing a cholangiogram, even if it is the CBD, it would be diagnosed and immediately repair even laparoscopically. On the contrary, if the misinterpretation continues, the false CD (CBD) is sectioned and the BDI is extremely complex since it is not infrequent to concomitantly injure the RHA, given the close relationship it has with the CBD [30, 31].
- Hemorrhage: It is a risky situation to produce a BDI when pursuing hemostasis, especially when these maneuvers are blind o desperate. They can be generated by deliberated titanium clips insertions, or even worse through the use of cautery, which ultimately provokes more extensive injuries and determines a higher frequency of stenosis in the remote follow-up [32].

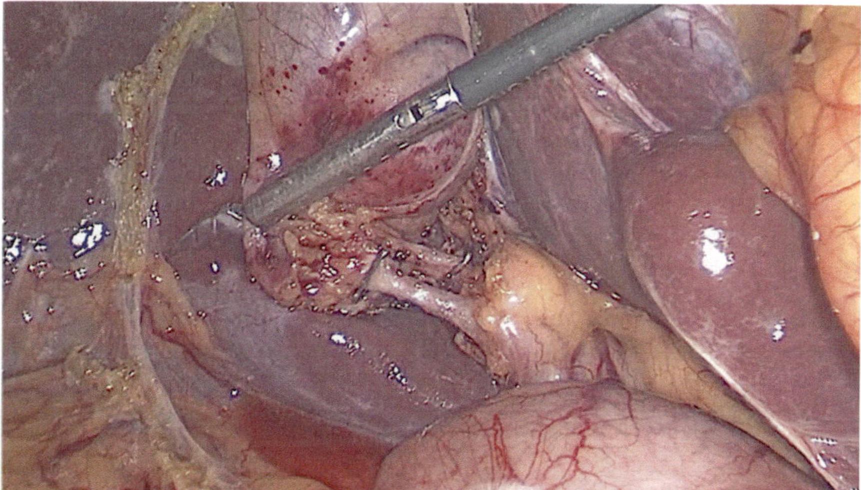

Fig. 5.1 "Strasberg's Critical View of Safety" Two structures (artery and cystic duct) can be seen reaching the gallbladder after dissection of the lower third of the gallbladder [29]

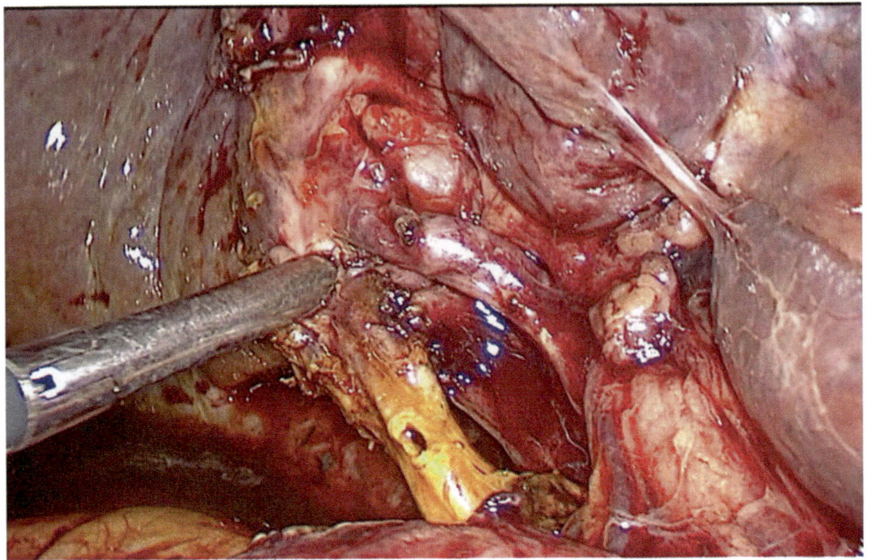

Fig. 5.2 Injury to Common Bile Duct (CBD) through a sharp section with scissors for cholangiography. Resection was avoided due to intraoperative diagnosis. The injury was repaired laparoscopically by an experienced surgeon

At this point, it is important to recognize the type of injury:

1. Cold section: The injury is committed by sharp instruments (scissors, scalpels, puncture instruments). As there is no thermal mechanism involved, the injury is limited to the area where the sectioning was performed. In other words, a primary repair at the level of the injury is usually sufficient, Fig. 5.2.
2. Cautery section: Thermal injuries were mainly introduced with the initiation of laparoscopic surgery. This type of injury, as it involves energy, is not limited to the damaged area. The necrotic process, due to inflammation or ischemia associated with monopolar energy, gradually progresses over the following days and weeks. All attempts of repair at this level are probably set to fail. In this case, it is advisable to call in an expert surgeon and to resect more extensively the injured area, or to postpone repair until it is well demarcated by progressive necrosis over time [33, 34].

All these factors previously described determine the characteristics of BDI in the laparoscopic era [35]:

- The majority are not recognized intraoperatively.
- The level of injury is higher than in the open approach (Strasberg E2, E3, E4) [36].
- A *thermal mechanism* is usually involved in the generation of the BDI.
- Frequently presents with an external biliary fistula, which results in a thin bile duct at the time of repair.

Conclusions

The causes and mechanisms of BDI are diverse. These will depend on different factors, dependent or independent of the patient. Recognition of the cause, mechanism, and type of injury is necessary to assess the type and timing of a definitive repair, all decisions that are determinant to achieve the best possible outcome.

References

1. Shallaly GEI, Cuschieri A. Nature, etiology and outcome of bile duct injuries after laparoscopic cholecystectomy. HPB. 2000;2:3–12.
2. Strasberg SM, Hertl M, Soper NJ. An analysis of the problem of biliary injury during laparoscopic cholecystectomy. J Am Coll Surg. 1995;180:101–25.
3. Marakis GN, Pavlidis TE, Ballas K, Aimoniotou E, Psarras K, Karvounaris D, Rafailidis S, Demertzidis H, Sakantamis AK. Major complications during laparoscopic cholecystectomy. Int Surg. 2007;92:142–6.
4. Michael Brunt L, Deziel DJ, Telem DA, et al. Safe cholecystectomy multi-society practice guideline and state-of-the-art consensus conference on prevention of bile duct injury during cholecystectomy. Surg Endosc. 2020;34:2827–55.
5. Perneger TV. The Swiss cheese model of safety incidents: are there holes in the metaphor? BMC Health Serv Res. 2005;5:71.
6. Marinov LM. The Mirizzi syndrome—a major cause for biliary duct injury during laparoscopic cholecystectomy. Biomed J Sci Tech Res. 2017. https://doi.org/10.26717/bjstr.2017.01.000308.
7. Greyasov VI, Chuguevsky VM, Sivokon NI, Agapov MA, Abubakarov RS. [Non-functioning gallbladder as a risk factor for bile ducts injury during laparoscopic cholecystectomy]. Khirurgiia. 2018;52–56.
8. Borzellino G, Sauerland S, Minicozzi AM, Verlato G, Di Pietrantonj C, de Manzoni G, Cordiano C. Laparoscopic cholecystectomy for severe acute cholecystitis. A meta-analysis of results. Surg Endosc. 2008;22:8–15.
9. Aziz H, Pandit V, Joseph B, Jie T, Ong E. Age and obesity are independent predictors of bile duct injuries in patients undergoing laparoscopic cholecystectomy. World J Surg. 2015;39:1804–8.
10. Bujanda L, Calvo MM, Cabriada JL, Orive V, Capelastegui A. MRCP in the diagnosis of iatrogenic bile duct injury. NMR Biomed. 2003;16:475–8.
11. Yeh TS, Jan YY, Tseng JH, Hwang TL, Jeng LB, Chen MF. Value of magnetic resonance cholangiopancreatography in demonstrating major bile duct injuries following laparoscopic cholecystectomy. Br J Surg. 1999;86:181–4.
12. Aduna M, Larena JA, Martín D, Martínez-Guereñu B, Aguirre I, Astigarraga E. Bile duct leaks after laparoscopic cholecystectomy: value of contrast-enhanced MRCP. Abdom Imaging. 2005;30:480–7.
13. Debru E, Dawson A, Leibman S, Richardson M, Glen L, Hollinshead J, Falk GL. Does routine intraoperative cholangiography prevent bile duct transection? Surg Endosc. 2005;19:589–93.
14. Christou N, Roux-David A, Naumann DN, et al. Bile duct injury during cholecystectomy: necessity to learn how to do and interpret intraoperative cholangiography. Front Med. 2021;8:637987.
15. Ankersmit M, van Dam DA, van Rijswijk A-S, van den Heuvel B, Tuynman JB, Meijerink WJHJ. Fluorescent imaging with indocyanine green during laparoscopic cholecystectomy in patients at increased risk of bile duct injury. Surg Innov. 2017;24:245–52.
16. Strasberg SM. Avoidance of biliary injury during laparoscopic cholecystectomy. J Hepatobiliary Pancreat Surg. 2002;9:543–7.

17. McKinley SK, Brunt LM, Schwaitzberg SD. Prevention of bile duct injury: the case for incorporating educational theories of expertise. Surg Endosc. 2014;28:3385–91.
18. Massarweh NN, Devlin A, Symons RG, Broeckel Elrod JA, Flum DR. Risk tolerance and bile duct injury: surgeon characteristics, risk-taking preference, and common bile duct injuries. J Am Coll Surg. 2009;209:17–24.
19. Calvete J, Sabater L, Camps B, Verdú A, Gomez-Portilla A, Martín J, Torrico MA, Flor B, Cassinello N, Lledó S. Bile duct injury during laparoscopic cholecystectomy: myth or reality of the learning curve? Surg Endosc. 2000;14:608–11.
20. Way LW, Stewart L, Gantert W, Liu K, Lee CM, Whang K, Hunter JG. Causes and prevention of laparoscopic bile duct injuries: analysis of 252 cases from a human factors and cognitive psychology perspective. Ann Surg. 2003;237:460–9.
21. Strasberg SM, Helton WS. An analytical review of vasculobiliary injury in laparoscopic and open cholecystectomy. HPB. 2011;13:1–14.
22. De Santibáñes E, Ardiles V, Pekolj J. Complex bile duct injuries: management. HPB. 2008;10:4–12.
23. Keleman AM, Imagawa DK, Findeiss L, et al. Associated vascular injury in patients with bile duct injury during cholecystectomy. Am Surg. 2011;77:1330–3.
24. Kaushik R. Bleeding complications in laparoscopic cholecystectomy: incidence, mechanisms, prevention and management. J Minim Access Surg. 2010;6:59–65.
25. Usal H, Sayad P, Hayek N, Hallak A, Huie F, Ferzli G. Major vascular injuries during laparoscopic cholecystectomy. An institutional review of experience with 2589 procedures and literature review. Surg Endosc. 1998;12:960–2.
26. Gupta V, Gupta V, Joshi P, Kumar S, Kulkarni R, Chopra N, Pavankumar G, Chandra A. Management of post cholecystectomy vascular injuries. Surgeon. 2019;17:326–33.
27. Caratozzolo E, Massani M, Recordare A, Bonariol L, Antoniutti M, Jelmoni A, Bassi N. Usefulness of both operative cholangiography and conversion to decrease major bile duct injuries during laparoscopic cholecystectomy. J Hepatobiliary Pancreat Surg. 2004;11:171–5.
28. Eikermann M, Siegel R, Broeders I, et al. Prevention and treatment of bile duct injuries during laparoscopic cholecystectomy: the clinical practice guidelines of the European Association for Endoscopic Surgery (EAES). Surg Endosc. 2012;26:3003–39.
29. Strasberg SM, Brunt LM. Rationale and use of the critical view of safety in laparoscopic cholecystectomy. J Am Coll Surg. 2010;211:132–8.
30. Renz BW, Bösch F, Angele MK. Bile duct injury after cholecystectomy: surgical therapy. Visc Med. 2017;33:184–90.
31. Strasberg SM, Gouma DJ. “Extreme” vasculobiliary injuries: association with fundus-down cholecystectomy in severely inflamed gallbladders. HPB. 2012;14:1–8.
32. Suuronen S, Kivivuori A, Tuimala J, Paajanen H. Bleeding complications in cholecystectomy: a register study of over 22,000 cholecystectomies in Finland. BMC Surg. 2015;15:97.
33. Nechay T, Sazhin A, Titkova S, Anurov M, Tyagunov A, Sheptunov S, Yakhutlov U, Nakhushev R, Sannikov A. Thermal processes in bile ducts during laparoscopic cholecystectomy with monopolar instruments. experimental study using real-time intraluminal and surface thermography. Surg Innov. 2021;28:525–35.
34. Portella AOV, Trindade MRM, Dias LZ, Goldenberg S, Trindade EN. Monopolar electrosurgery on the extrahepatic bile ducts during laparoscopic cholecystectomy: an experimental controlled trial. Surg Laparosc Endosc Percutan Tech. 2009;19:213–6.
35. Hogan NM, Dorcaratto D, Hogan AM, Nasirawan F, McEntee P, Maguire D, Geoghegan J, Traynor O, Winter DC, Hoti E. Iatrogenic common bile duct injuries: increasing complexity in the laparoscopic era: a prospective cohort study. Int J Surg. 2016;33 Pt A:151–6.
36. Stewart L. Iatrogenic biliary injuries: identification, classification, and management. Surg Clin North Am. 2014;94:297–310.

Chapter 6
Classification of BDI

David Alberto Biagiola, Ignacio Merlo, Juan Glinka, and Rodrigo Sanchez Clária

Introduction

The aim of classifying DBI is to formulate unified concepts that would permit the collection of data useful for comparative studies and consolidate specific treatments for each type of lesion.

The description of BDI's also evolved with experience and technological development. Nowadays, the understanding of the specific mechanism of BDI and its

D. A. Biagiola
HPB Surgery and Liver Transplant Unit, Sanatorio Parque, Rosario, Argentina

I. Merlo
General Surgery Service, Hospital Italiano de Buenos Aires, Buenos Aires, Argentina

J. Glinka
Division of HPB Surgery and Multiorgan Transplant Unit, Western University – London Regional Cancer Program, London, ON, Canada

R. S. Clária (✉)
HPB Surgery and Intestinal Transplant Unit, Hospital Italiano de Buenos Aires, Buenos Aires, Argentina
e-mail: rodrigo.sanchez@hospitalitaliano.org.ar

J. Pekolj et al. (eds.), *Fundamentals of Bile Duct Injuries*, https://doi.org/10.1007/978-3-031-13383-1_6

consequences is granted by the numerous high-fidelity studies that are routinely available [1].

Moreover, the higher incidence of BDI over the last three decades (since the implementation of laparoscopic surgery) provided a cumulative experience that ultimately facilitates the comprehension of this pathology and more precise and a thorough classification.

However, the most comprehensive classification systems were not widely adopted, and the international community still prefers the traditional descriptions. This could be explained by the fact that the simplest classifications have a better transdisciplinary adoption. In other words, it is easier to communicate with our colleagues from disciplines other than surgery treating BDIs together (gastroenterologists, endoscopists, interventional and non-interventional radiologists, etc.) using simpler classifications.

Therefore, in this section we aim to provide a multidisciplinary overview of these simplest and yet most commonly used classifications of BDIs [2].

Bismuth Classification

In 1982, Prof. Henri Bismuth described the first anatomical classification to delineate the severity of a postoperative biliary stenosis based on the height of the injury in the biliary tree. Determining the level of the BDI using the IOC permitted the selection of the most appropriate surgical strategy for a successful repair. It is also utilized to classify tumors of the main bile ducts according to their location [3].

This classification is extremely simple, was rapidly adopted, and is still in use, Fig. 6.1.

→

Fig. 6.1 Bismuth classification. ***Type I*** *When the injury involves the Common Bile Duct (CBD) at least 2 cm below the confluence of the hepatic ducts.* ***Type II*** *When the injury involves the CBD at less than 2 cm of the confluence of the hepatic ducts.* ***Type III*** *Hilar injury/stricture with preserved biliary confluence at both sides.* ***Type IV*** *Hilar injury/stricture with destruction of the confluence: the right and left hepatic ducts are separated.* ***Type V*** *Involves an aberrant right hepatic duct with or without injury of the CBD*

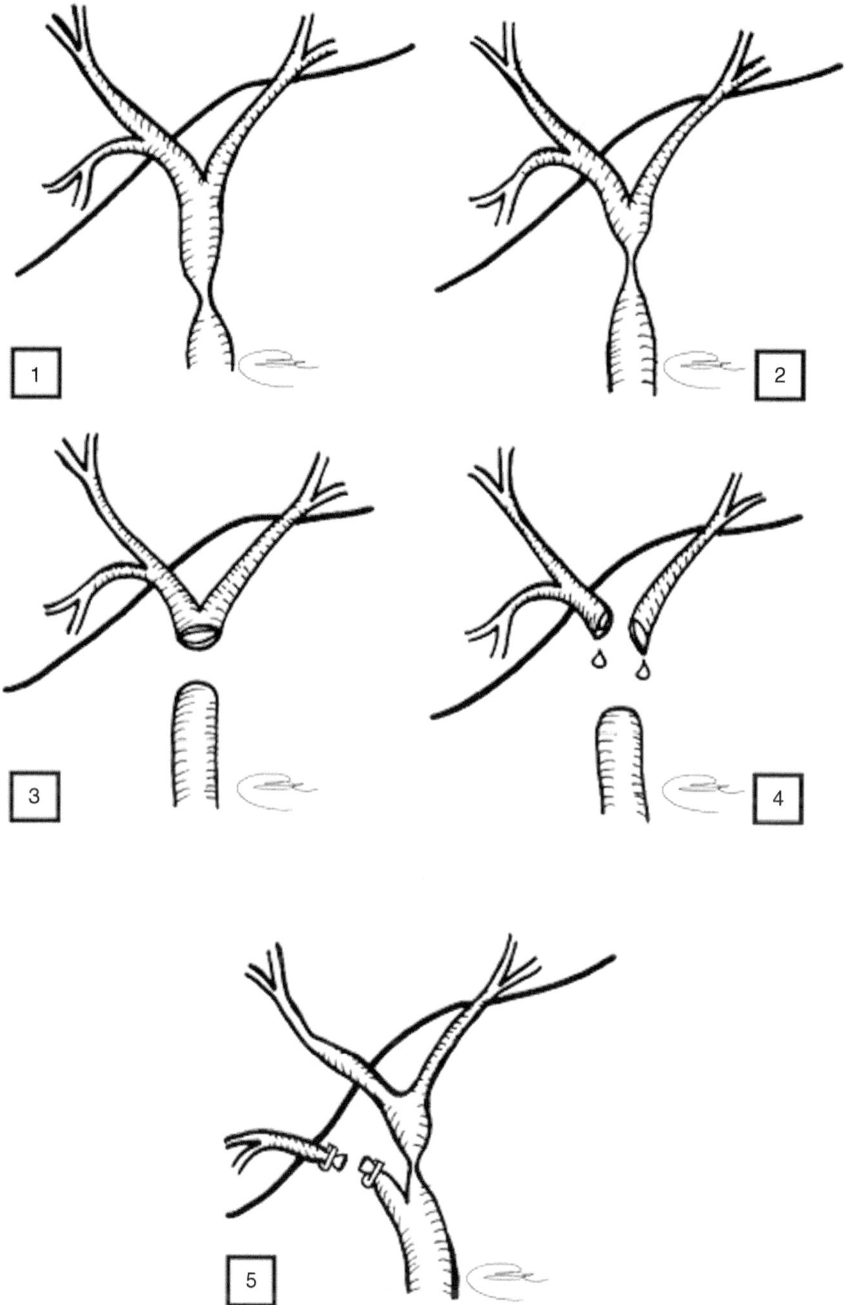
1
2
3
4
5

Strasberg Classification

The Strasberg classification (Fig. 6.2) is more comprehensive as it allows differentiation between *minor injuries*, such as bile leakage from the CD or an aberrant right posterior duct (RHD), from more severe injuries [4, 5]. It is a very simple classification as well and can be easily comprehended and the different grades are as follows:

- ***Type A****: Is a bile leak from the CD or the liver bed without CBD injury?*

  Bile leakage from the cystic duct can occur due to failure of CD ligation, which may be secondary to increased intrabiliary pressure generated by untreated intracoledochal lithiasis, or migration of titanium clips causing a leak.

  Bile leakage from the liver bed is frequently due to dissection in the wrong deep plane resulting in the injury of small peripheral ducts called "subvesicular bile ducts," mainly tributary to the RHD. These are also controversially named as Luschka's ducts, although some authors believe that these are different accessory bile ducts that may communicate the main intrahepatic bile ducts with the gallbladder [6, 7] [*see* Chap. 2].

  Although this biliary leak can be life threatening if left untreated, in our daily practice it is not considered a genuine BDI. Our assertion is based on the fact that these leaks are not accompanied by the serious problems and the uncertainty that accompanies true injuries of the main biliary duct: the potential for developing biliary stenosis and its consequent cholestasis.
- ***Type B***: *Occlusion of the aberrant right hepatic duct.* It manifests with late postoperative pain, cholangitis, or may be completely asymptomatic.
- ***Type C***: *This represents a bile leak from a BDI including fistula by proximal section of the aberrant right hepatic duct that is not in communication with the CBD.* Type C injuries manifest with initial postoperative pain, fever, or sepsis secondary to the bile leak conditioning a biloma and/or peritonitis. Imaging studies usually identify an intra-abdominal biliary collection. *Endoscopic Retrograde Cholangiopancreatography (ERCP) shows no evidence of radiopaque contrast leakage, as the area of leakage is not connected to the main biliary duct* [8].
- ***Type D***: These are lateral injuries of the extrahepatic bile ducts. In these injuries, there is a loss of substance of less than 50% of the circumference of the biliary tree.
- ***Type E:*** Replicate Bismuth's classification in which there is a loss of continuity of the biliary tree, either by stenosis, complete occlusion (ligation or clipping), resection (with loss of substance), or thermal injury of the hepatic ducts or main biliary duct. Strasberg E lesions are subsequently divided—*in a similar way as Bismuth classification*—into:

  E1: CBD injury >2 cm distal to the biliary confluence.
  E2: CBD injury <2 cm from the biliary confluence.
  E3: Hilar stricture with the right and left ducts in communication.
  E4: Hilar stricture with separation of right and left ducts.
  E5: Stricture of the CBD and the aberrant RHD.

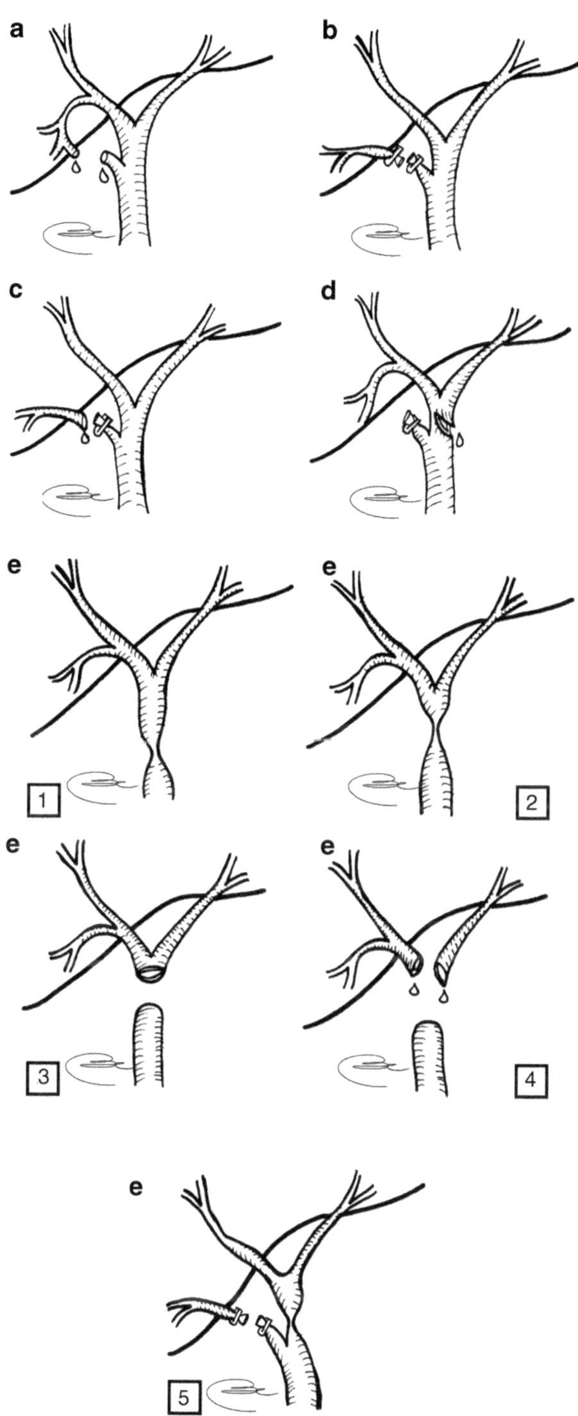

Fig. 6.2 Strasberg's classification

The main disadvantage of both Strasberg's and Bismuth's classifications is that they do not include associated vascular compromise, which is extremely important in decision-making and prognosis.

Stewart–Way Classification

The Stewart–Way classification provides insight and understanding of the mechanism of injury by considering biliary injury and concomitant vascular lesions (Fig. 6.3).

This is a more complex classification that provides useful information on the pathophysiology of BDI. This is a more complex classification that provides thorough information on the pathophysiology of BDI. As a result, it helps in understanding more precisely how the injuries occurred which would also be of use to developing preventive mechanisms to reduce their incidence. In addition, it differentiates between injuries that resect segments of the biliary duct and those that generate stenosis, which is useful for guiding preoperative evaluation and determining a surgical strategy for future biliary reconstructions. Even though it is a comprehensive classification and can be challenging to embrace, we believe it is helpful in predicting the mechanism of injury and, as we mentioned, elaborate prevention strategies [9, 10].

This classification divides biliary duct injuries into four types I, II (A, B, C, D), III (A, B, C, D), and IV as follows:

- ***Type I*** (6% of cases) consists of a partial incision *(without a complete section)* of the CBD.

  It occurs when CBD is mistaken for the cystic duct, but the error is recognized through a cholangiogram before CBD is divided [11, 12].
- ***Type II*** (24% of cases) consists of an injury to CBD from clips or thermal injury applied near the duct. This frequently occurs in challenging cases where visibility is limited due to inflammation or trying to resolve a bleeding. Is not infrequent to observe in the imaging the presence of numerous metallic clips attempting blind hemostatic maneuvers on this type of lesions.
- ***Type III*** (60% of cases) is the most common type and consists of a complete transection at a variable portion of the CBD. These injuries result from misperception of the common bile duct as a cystic duct, and most of the time the anatomy is not confirmed by an IOC.
- ***Type II and III injuries*** *are further subdivided according to the proximal extent of the injury into A, B, C, and D:*

Fig. 6.3 Stewart–Way classification

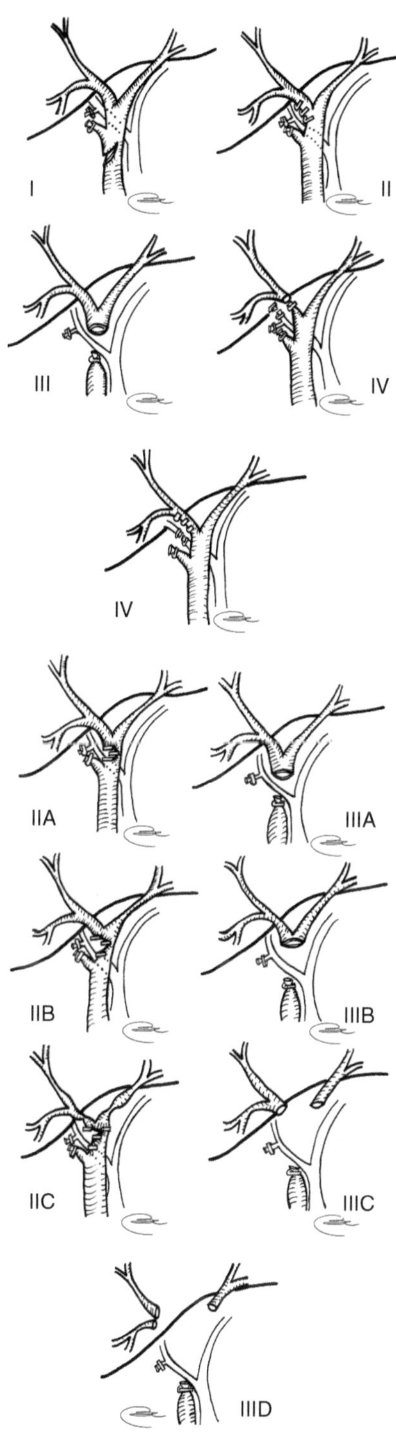

Type II–III A*: Preserves the confluence of the hepatic ducts and some CBD at variable degrees.*

Type II–III B*: Involves section or stenosis at the confluence of the CBD.*

Type II–III C*: Result from stenosis or extended resection of the biliary tree above the confluence of the right and left hepatic ducts.*

Type III D*: (not seen in type II) Results from section and loss of substance above the first bifurcation of the lobar ducts. It is rare and results from following the extrahepatic biliary tree into the hilar space with excision of all extrahepatic ducts.*

- **Type IV** injuries (10% of cases) involve damage (resection or stenosis) of the RHD either normal or aberrant. It is frequently associated (60% of cases) with an injury to the right hepatic artery (RHA). The injuries are caused by misidentification of the RHD (or an aberrant right duct) as the CD and the RHA as the cystic artery; or from lateral injury of the RHD (or aberrant) during dissection of Calot's triangle.

Conclusions

Even though there are more than a dozen different classifications, the ones discussed in this section are the most used in everyday practice mainly based on their simplicity and their transdisciplinary acceptance.

These are helpful to determine the anatomical level the of injury based on the BDI description and orient the therapeutic efforts accordingly. With Stewart and Way's classification, it is possible to infer the physiopathology of the injury as well, therefore it seems great to understand the context in which a BDI occurs and subsequently elaborate prevention strategies [13].

It should be noted that these classification systems, since they are anatomical and descriptive, do not incorporate key clinical information such as the patient's condition (sepsis, hemodynamic decompensation, etc.) the time of injury recognition, all of which significantly influence the management strategy, and obviously the outcome.

References

1. Mercado MA, Domínguez I. Classification and management of bile duct injuries. World J Gastrointest Surg. 2011;3:43–8.
2. Bektas H, Schrem H, Winny M, Klempnauer J. Surgical treatment and outcome of iatrogenic bile duct lesions after cholecystectomy and the impact of different clinical classification systems. Br J Surg. 2007;94:1119–27.
3. Bismuth H. Postoperative strictures of the bile ducts. In: Blumgart LH, editor. The Biliary Tract V. New York, NY: Churchill-Livingstone; 1982. pp. 209–18.

4. Strasberg SM, Hertl M, Soper NJ. An analysis of the problem of biliary injury during laparoscopic cholecystectomy. J Am Coll Surg. 1995;180:101–25.
5. Strasberg SM, Picus DD, Drebin JA. Results of a new strategy for reconstruction of biliary injuries having an isolated right-sided component. J Gastrointest Surg. 2001;5:266–74.
6. Spanos CP, Syrakos T. Bile leaks from the duct of Luschka (subvesical duct): a review. Langenbecks Arch Surg. 2006;391:441–7.
7. Iida H, Matsui Y, Kaibori M, Matsui K, Ishizaki M, Hamada H, Kon M. Single-center experience with subvesical bile ducts (ducts of Luschka). Am Surg. 2017;83:e43–5.
8. Yeh TS, Jan YY, Tseng JH, Hwang TL, Jeng LB, Chen MF. Value of magnetic resonance cholangiopancreatography in demonstrating major bile duct injuries following laparoscopic cholecystectomy. Br J Surg. 1999;86:181–4.
9. Stewart L, Way LW. Bile duct injuries during laparoscopic cholecystectomy. Factors that influence the results of treatment. Arch Surg. 1995;130:1123–8; discussion 1129.
10. Stewart L, Way LW. Laparoscopic bile duct injuries: timing of surgical repair does not influence success rate. A multivariate analysis of factors influencing surgical outcomes. HPB. 2009;11:516–22.
11. Debru E, Dawson A, Leibman S, Richardson M, Glen L, Hollinshead J, Falk GL. Does routine intraoperative cholangiography prevent bile duct transection? Surg Endosc. 2005;19:589–93.
12. Alvarez FA, de Santibañes M, Palavecino M, Sánchez Clariá R, Mazza O, Arbues G, de Santibañes E, Pekolj J. Impact of routine intraoperative cholangiography during laparoscopic cholecystectomy on bile duct injury. Br J Surg. 2014;101:677–84.
13. Michael Brunt L, Deziel DJ, Telem DA, et al. Safe cholecystectomy multi-society practice guideline and state-of-the-art consensus conference on prevention of bile duct injury during cholecystectomy. Surg Endosc. 2020;34:2827–55.

Chapter 7
Intraoperative Diagnosis and Treatment

Martin Palavecino

Introduction

BDI is still the most undesirable complication of laparoscopic cholecystectomy (LC) [1].

Contrary to the expectations, during the introduction of the laparoscopic approach, the incidence did not decrease but rather increased. In most series, it remains between 0.3 and 0.5% while in conventional surgery it was 0.2%. Long-term poor prognostic outcomes occur when there is a late diagnosis of the injury, or when there are several unsuccessful attempts of repair, usually by surgeons inexperienced in complex biliary pathology [2].

Unfortunately, the mortality rate may reach 7% when the injuries are complex and/or with late complications. In some cases, it can even lead to terminal liver disease, requiring a liver transplant (LT) as the ultimate measure [3].

Intraoperative diagnosis of a BDI is the ideal moment to prevent late diagnosis complications (cholangitis, bilomas, choleperitoneum, etc.). At the same time, it enables immediate and definitive repair, usually by laparoscopic approach, by trained surgeons, and significantly reduces the rate of malpractice claims [4].

Although it is widely agreed that these patients should be treated by expert surgeons, the best timing of repair strategy is still controversial for some authors and depends primarily on the experience of the treating medical team. Recent studies, including those conducted at the Hospital Italiano de Buenos Aires, demonstrate that immediate intraoperative repair performed by surgeons trained in complex biliary surgery is significantly associated with low morbidity and excellent long-term results [4, 5]. Zero tolerance of BDI is desirable, although difficult to achieve, this

M. Palavecino (✉)
HPB Surgery, General Surgery Service, Hospital Italiano de San Justo, Prov Buenos Aires, Argentina
e-mail: martin.palavecino@hospitalitaliano.org.ar

J. Pekolj et al. (eds.), *Fundamentals of Bile Duct Injuries*,
https://doi.org/10.1007/978-3-031-13383-1_7

has led a group in the UK to create a specialized mobile biliary surgeon service, with specialists visiting the hospital where the bile duct injury occurred and performing the repair during the same procedure [6].

This policy offers an additional benefit since the surgeon who performs the repair is different from the surgeon who performed the injury, an optimal situation as it prevents the negative effects of discovering that a surgical injury to the bile duct has been performed by the operating surgeon himself [7].

In this chapter, the aspects to be considered in the intraoperative diagnosis of a bile duct injury will be described, and immediate treatment algorithms will be discussed during the actual surgery.

Intraoperative Diagnosis

Even though this is the ideal diagnosis, and secondary prevention should ideally focus on this, most publications worldwide still show results that are different from what is expected. Only 15–30% of injuries are diagnosed during surgery [8].

As aforementioned previously, the advantages of intraoperative diagnosis are:

- Avoiding complications and organic sequelae resulting from late diagnosis.
- Enabling appropriate steps for delayed definitive correction or immediate repair if an experienced surgeon is present.
- Reducing the high costs resulting from chronic treatment.
- Reducing legal disputes resulting from patients' or their environment's dissatisfaction.

Intraoperative diagnosis may occur in two forms:

1. Directly: By the surgeon's direct detection of the injury in the presence of transection of a previously unrecognized duct or by the presence of a bile leak.
2. Indirectly: Through abnormal findings (dye leak or loss of continuity of ducts in any sector of the intrahepatic or extrahepatic biliary tree) during Intraoperative Cholangiogram (IOC), Fig. 7.1.

In the event of direct detection, the injuries often occur by chance, especially when the patient has anatomical variants or partial stenosis secondary to the placement of clips in the proximity of the bile duct. In indirect diagnosis, i.e., by IOC, several publications have already established that this tool does not prevent BDI, but it has been demonstrated that they are less serious, more distal to the biliary confluent, and generally performed by cold section, without the use of electrocautery (with the consequences that this involves). The minor severity of these lesions encourages the surgeon to pause at the injury, avoid aggravating the injury (usually by transecting or extending the dissection and devascularization, or by adding an arterial or portal vascular injury), refer to a more experienced and/or non-emotionally involved surgeon, and proceed with the surgery, if possible, by repairing the injury [9].

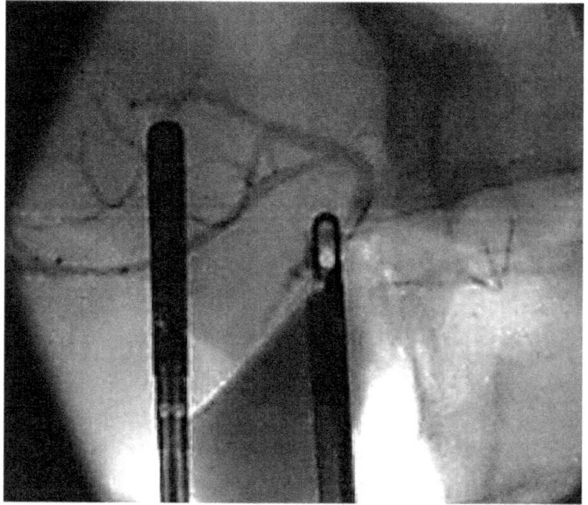

Fig. 7.1 Lateral injury of the right posterior hepatic duct. Olsen's clamp is holding the catheter inserted only in the injured duct. Contrast leakage into the abdominal cavity is observed

Nevertheless, there is still debate in literature and at scientific conventions events as to whether IOC should be considered a standard of care and should be performed systematically or whether it should be an optional procedure according to the discretion of the surgical medical team [10]. At the Hospital Italiano de Buenos Aires, IOC is routinely performed, since the days of open surgery. This enables residency training in Cystic Duct (CD) cannulation, interpretation of normal anatomy and anatomical variants, as well as laparoscopic exploration of the CBD if required. Therefore, the incidence of BDI in this series was 0.17%, which is even lower than most of the publications. Ninety percent of the injuries were diagnosed intraoperatively and most were mild lesions (75% Strasberg D type lesions) and there were no associated vascular injuries. The two injuries that were not diagnosed intraoperatively (10%) were non-transmural electrocautery injuries, resulting in late perforation and stenosis. While IOC may have a greater protective effect in high-risk patients (men and patients with acute cholecystitis), the selective use of IOC is, however, not recommended considering that up to 50% of BID occurs in patients without risk factors [11].

Arguments supporting the systematic use of CIO include:

- A decrease in the incidence of BDI.
- Prevention of serious injuries.
- Increased intraoperative detection.
- Lower morbidity and mortality rates.
- Diagnosis and treatment of unsuspected choledochal lithiasis.

Besides, the systematic use of IOC provides an adequate learning curve for the surgeon and the rest of the treating medical team, planning significantly reduces operating times, and improving surgical skills for CBD exploration. The surgeon's greater knowledge of anatomical variations reduces the misinterpretation of images, especially during residency training. Whereas an estimated 500–700 IOC are required to prevent just one late-diagnosed BID, it is a proven patient benefit and financially cost-effective practice, as the cost of treatment in a late-diagnosed patient may be up to 16 times higher than the total cost of a combined IOC and immediate repair [12, 13].

Intraoperative Management and Repair Techniques

The type and duration of repair of a BDI will depend on several factors:

- Time of diagnosis of the injury (noticed during primary surgery or unnoticed).
- Type of injury (using some of the classical classifications: Strasberg [14], Bismuth [15], Stewart & Way [16]) (See Chap. 6).
- Mechanism of injury (clipping, ligation, section with cold scissors, use of electrocautery).
- Experience of the treating surgeon.

When the injuries correspond to partial, small, and cold mechanism sections with a fine biliary duct, as is usually the case in partial sections with scissors for IOC, the recommendation is to perform direct suturing with delicate threads and to place abdominal drains in the area. This repair can be performed laparoscopically, with the advantages of laparoscopy such as good exposure and magnification. In such cases, the placement of an external biliary drain (T-Tube) may involve more biliary damage than benefit. This would be comparable to cases of small tears of the CD/CBD junction in open surgery, in which only separated stitches and an abdominal drain are placed due to the risk of postoperative bile leak [17]. If a T-Tube is necessary, it can also be replaced by a transpapillary plastic prosthesis placed laparoscopically and then removed endoscopically, Fig. 7.2.

In situations where the section is total, but without resection of the bile duct and if the damage was performed without the use of electrocoagulation, the

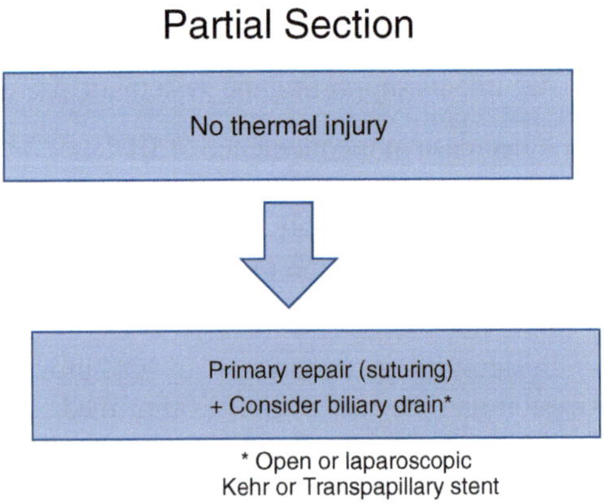

Fig. 7.2 Partial section algorithm

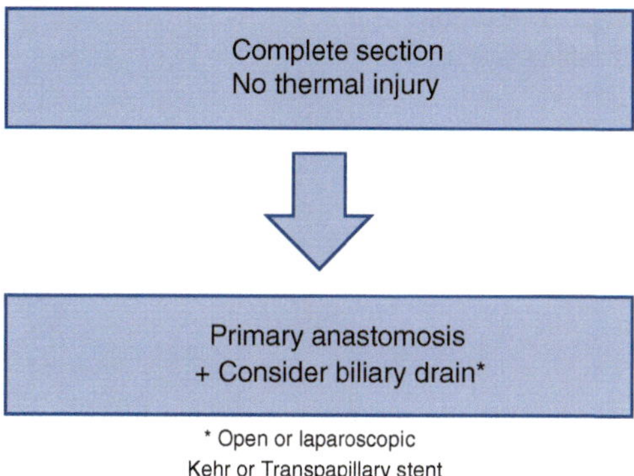

Fig. 7.3 Total section algorithm

recommendation is to perform an end-to-end suture of the CBD as far as no tension exists between the ends, placing a T-Tube above or below the injury. Whereas in many cases there may be partial scissor injuries where there was no thermal mechanism, other factors such as excessive dissection (due to anatomical misinterpretation) may also cause local ischemia and should be considered in the decision to repair [18, 19], Fig. 7.3.

In the case of thermal injuries, such injuries take time to be evident due to their progressive extension, and therefore, the classic recommendation, in surgeons without experience in the management of this type of situation, is to delay treatment (by placing drains and referring the patient to a referral center).

When the diagnosis is established intraoperatively and experienced surgeons are available, the proximal bile duct needs to be resected until a thin, healthy-walled, and well-irrigated duct. Upon completion, a Roux-en-Y hepaticojejunostomy (RYHJ) reconstruction should be performed [20]. This repair should be conducted by an experienced surgeon, as it is usually a non-dilated bile duct, which requires the use of magnification (magnifying glasses) to perform an adequate plastic repair without postoperative stenosis (usually separate stitches of resorbable material) [21].

As in cases of thermal damage, the ideal surgery for bile duct resection is a RYHJ. Repair using the duodenum is not recommended for two main reasons: in the first place, both because it is not an ideal reconstruction (it does not exclude intestinal transit) and in second place because in the event of an anastomotic biliary fistula, a lateral duodenal fistula would be added as well. Furthermore, in young patients, it should be considered that biliary-digestive bypasses using the duodenum have a 4-times higher risk of developing malignant biliary neoplasms after 10 years than those performed with a RYHJ [22], Fig. 7.4.

The advantages of repair performed by experienced surgeons during the same surgery in which the injury was committed are:

- Definitive repair during the same surgery and the positive impact this has on the patient and his/her family.
- Avoiding referring the patient to another institution.

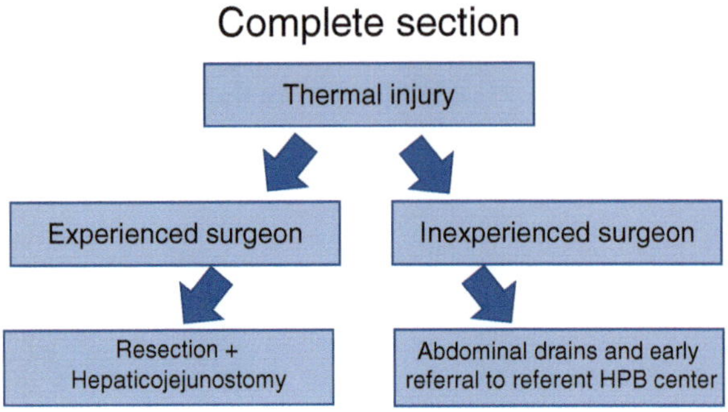

Fig. 7.4 Resection and/or thermal injury algorithm

Complete section

Thermal injury

Experienced surgeon → Resection + Hepaticojejunostomy

Inexperienced surgeon → Abdominal drains and early referral to referent HPB center

- Shorter hospital stays.
- Less abdominal and biliary drainage.
- Less psychological trauma on the patient and, therefore less probability of legal action.

Concerning the procedure for the repair of a surgical injury of the bile duct, it can be open or laparoscopic depending on the complexity, the type of injury, and the surgeon's experience and training level. At Hospital Italiano, one-third of the autogenous injuries diagnosed at surgery were successfully repaired without changing converting to conventional surgery. Laparoscopic repair is possible if the injuries are limited, with non-thermal mechanism, and the surgeon has experience in advanced laparoscopic techniques. Under these circumstances, magnification and delicate laparoscopic instrumentation may be advantageous for the skilled surgeon.

Frequently, the surgeon causing a BDI during LC has no experience in the management of this complication and further damage or delay may occur. Therefore, when the surgeon is not properly qualified or trained or does not have the necessary equipment and the possibility to be supported immediately by a specialist, the surgeon should only be concerned about placing a drain in the bile duct and some in the subhepatic area to avoid possible collections or a coleperitoneum that may require an early reoperation. Once the patient is stabilized, he/she should be transferred to a referral center with experience in this type of repair to provide better, long-term results [23, 24].

Further dissection of the bile duct and ligation of the bile duct is not recommended so as to avoid the risk of cholangitis. The purpose of this scenario is to stay away from three major complications: coleperitoneum, localized biliary collections, and cholangitis.

The risks of proceeding with surgery without the necessary experience include a further extension of the injury, the sacrifice of vital tissues, and damage to vascular structures, mainly the right hepatic artery (RHA). These factors further complicate the prognosis. If the surgeon notices a significant injury, he/she can place the subhepatic drains laparoscopically rather than turning the patient, preventing further potential parietal complications [25].

Outcomes of Repairs in the Same Surgical Procedure

The most recent publications describing the repair in the same surgical procedure for bile duct injury have reported an effectiveness of 85–89%. They also demonstrate that immediate repair by skilled surgeons provides long-term results comparable to delayed repair (with similar rates of reoperation, recurrent cholangitis, or restenosis); fortunately, they have significantly less morbidity (half) [26, 27].

At the Hospital Italiano, morbidity and mortality in 17 patients who had intraoperative repair were 29% and 0%, respectively, with a median hospital stay of 6 days. In 15 patients (88.2%), the repair was successful and they had a favorable outcome. Only 2 patients (11.7%) had early biliary stenosis and were successfully treated secondarily with excellent results. In both cases, these were wrongly indicated as simple closures during the learning curve (thermal injury in one patient and ischemia due to devascularization in the other), with direct implications for the repair failure. After a median follow-up of 71 months (range 14–220 months), all patients had successful outcomes with normal clinical and alkaline phosphatase controls [5, 4].

Conclusions

IOC is an excellent tool both for early intraoperative detection of BDI and for the prevention of serious injuries. Intraoperative repair by skilled surgeons provides the least traumatic and the shortest route to achieve excellent long-term results in these patients.

In well-trained hands and in the presence of injuries that do not involve a thermal mechanism, it is advisable the injury repair (simple closure if it is a partial cut or anastomosis if it is a total cut) with or without the use of a T-tube or a transpapillary plastic prosthesis laparoscopically positioned. In cases of compromised vascularization (due to resection or thermal damage), it is advisable to resect the bile duct and to perform a RYHJ with a healthy bile duct. If the surgeon who caused the injury is not properly trained or has no possibility of being supported immediately by a specialist, he/she should exclusively place drains in the bile duct and subhepatic area and subsequently transfer the patient to a referral center with professionals who have experience in the management of this pathology, Fig. 7.5.

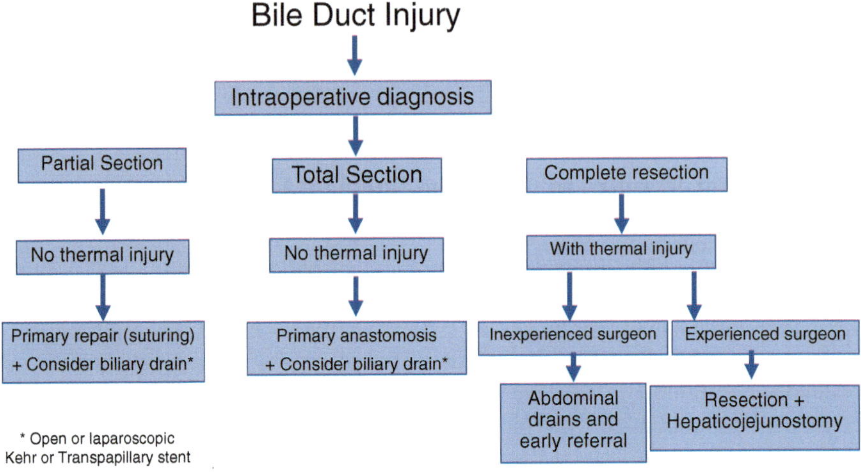

Fig. 7.5 Final algorithm

References

1. Shallaly GEI, Cuschieri A. Nature, aetiology and outcome of bile duct injuries after laparoscopic cholecystectomy. HPB. 2000;2:3–12.
2. Michael Brunt L, Deziel DJ, Telem DA, et al. Safe cholecystectomy multi-society practice guideline and state-of-the-art consensus conference on prevention of bile duct injury during cholecystectomy. Surg Endosc. 2020;34:2827–55.
3. Booij KAC, de Reuver PR, van Dieren S, van Delden OM, Rauws EA, Busch OR, van Gulik TM, Gouma DJ. Long-term impact of bile duct injury on morbidity, mortality, quality of life, and work related limitations. Ann Surg. 2018;268:143–50.
4. Pekolj J, Alvarez FA, Palavecino M, Sánchez Clariá R, Mazza O, de Santibañes E. Intraoperative management and repair of bile duct injuries sustained during 10,123 laparoscopic cholecystectomies in a high-volume referral center. J Am Coll Surg. 2013;216:894–901.
5. De Santibáñes E, Ardiles V, Pekolj J. Complex bile duct injuries: management. HPB. 2008;10:4–12.
6. Silva MA, Coldham C, Mayer AD, Bramhall SR, Buckels JAC, Mirza DF. Specialist outreach service for on-table repair of iatrogenic bile duct injuries--a new kind of "travelling surgeon". Ann R Coll Surg Engl. 2008;90:243–6.
7. Massarweh NN, Devlin A, Symons RG, Broeckel Elrod JA, Flum DR. Risk tolerance and bile duct injury: surgeon characteristics, risk-taking preference, and common bile duct injuries. J Am Coll Surg. 2009;209:17–24.
8. Rystedt JML, Montgomery AK. Quality-of-life after bile duct injury: intraoperative detection is crucial. A national case-control study HPB. 2016;18:1010–6.
9. Debru E, Dawson A, Leibman S, Richardson M, Glen L, Hollinshead J, Falk GL. Does routine intraoperative cholangiography prevent bile duct transection? Surg Endosc. 2005;19:589–93.
10. Ragulin-Coyne E, Witkowski ER, Chau Z, Ng SC, Santry HP, Callery MP, Shah SA, Tseng JF. Is routine intraoperative cholangiogram necessary in the twenty-first century? A national view. J Gastrointest Surg. 2013;17:434–42.
11. Alvarez FA, de Santibañes M, Palavecino M, Sánchez Clariá R, Mazza O, Arbues G, de Santibañes E, Pekolj J. Impact of routine intraoperative cholangiography during laparoscopic cholecystectomy on bile duct injury. Br J Surg. 2014;101:677–84.

12. Buddingh KT, Weersma RK, Savenije RAJ, van Dam GM, Nieuwenhuijs VB. Lower rate of major bile duct injury and increased intraoperative management of common bile duct stones after implementation of routine intraoperative cholangiography. J Am Coll Surg. 2011;213:267–74.
13. Wysocki AP. Population-based studies should not be used to justify a policy of routine cholangiography to prevent major bile duct injury during laparoscopic cholecystectomy. World J Surg. 2017;41:82–9.
14. Strasberg SM, Hertl M, Soper NJ. An analysis of the problem of biliary injury during laparoscopic cholecystectomy. J Am Coll Surg. 1995;180:101–25.
15. Bismuth H. Postoperative strictures of the bile duct. Biliary Tract Clin Surg Int. 1982;5:209–18.
16. Stewart L. Iatrogenic biliary injuries: identification, classification, and management. Surg Clin North Am. 2014;94:297–310.
17. Rystedt J, Lindell G, Montgomery A. Bile duct injuries associated with 55,134 cholecystectomies: treatment and outcome from a National Perspective. World J Surg. 2016;40:73–80.
18. Sicklick JK, Camp MS, Lillemoe KD, et al. Surgical management of bile duct injuries sustained during laparoscopic cholecystectomy: perioperative results in 200 patients. Ann Surg. 2005;241(786–92):discussion 793–5.
19. Bektas H, Schrem H, Winny M, Klempnauer J. Surgical treatment and outcome of iatrogenic bile duct lesions after cholecystectomy and the impact of different clinical classification systems. Br J Surg. 2007;94:1119–27.
20. Benkabbou A, Castaing D, Salloum C, Adam R, Azoulay D, Vibert E. Treatment of failed roux-en-Y hepaticojejunostomy after post-cholecystectomy bile ducts injuries. Surgery. 2013;153:95–102.
21. A European-African HepatoPancreatoBiliary Association (E-AHPBA) Research Collaborative Study management group, Other members of the European-African HepatoPancreatoBiliary Association Research Collaborative. Post cholecystectomy bile duct injury: early, intermediate or late repair with hepaticojejunostomy - an E-AHPBA multi-center study. HPB. 2019;21:1641–7.
22. Kapoor VK. Management of Bile Duct Injury Detected Intraoperatively. In: Kapoor VK, editor. Post-cholecystectomy bile duct injury. Singapore: Springer Singapore; 2020. p. 97–107.
23. Lindemann J, Krige JEJ, Kotze U, Jonas E. Factors leading to loss of patency after biliary reconstruction of major laparoscopic cholecystectomy bile duct injuries: an observational study with long-term outcomes. HPB. 2020;22:1613–21.
24. Walsh RM, Matthew Walsh R, Michael Henderson J, Vogt DP, Brown N. Long-term outcome of biliary reconstruction for bile duct injuries from laparoscopic cholecystectomies. Surgery. 2007;142:450–7.
25. Keleman AM, Imagawa DK, Findeiss L, et al. Associated vascular injury in patients with bile duct injury during cholecystectomy. Am Surg. 2011;77:1330–3.
26. Pekolj J, Drago J. Controversies in iatrogenic bile duct injuries. Role of video-assisted laparoscopy in the management of iatrogenic bile duct injuries. Cir Esp. 2020;98:61–3.
27. Drago J, de Santibañes M, Palavecino M, Sánchez Claría R, Arbúes G, Mazza O, Pekolj J. Role of laparoscopy in the immediate, intermediate, and long-term management of iatrogenicbile duct injuries during laparoscopic cholecystectomy. Langenbeck's Arch Surg. 2022;407(2):663–73.

Chapter 8
Postoperative Diagnosis of BDI's

Victoria Ardiles and David Alberto Biagiola

Introduction

BDI still poses a major issue worldwide. Most injuries occur during LC, which is one of the most commonly performed surgeries. Several studies have shown a decreasing rate not only in the quality of life but also in the long-term survival of those patients suffering from a BID [1, 2]. Furthermore, a reduction in work capacity, an increase in absenteeism, and greater disability have also been analyzed, with consequent economic implications [3].

It should also be brought to attention that in many cases these patients are young and with no other pathology associated. Moreover, a low-medium complexity surgery, from which the patient should recover rather quickly becomes a major event that risks the patient's life and leaves them with chronic sequelae [4].

However, correct initial management of patients may decrease the impact of this complication on morbidity and mortality, quality of life, and long-term survival [5].

Once BID has been produced, the ideal situation is to make the diagnosis in the same surgical act. Nevertheless, this occurs in a smaller percentage of cases (and is conditioned upon the surgeon's experience, the use or not of IOC, etc.) [6].

The *early* postoperative diagnosis then assumes a starring role, and if it is early and correct, allows the implementation of effective treatment, reducing short and long-term complications with the subsequent impact on survival and quality of life as well [7].

V. Ardiles (✉)
HPB Surgery and Liver Transplant Unit, Hospital Italiano de Buenos Aires, Buenos Aires, Argentina
e-mail: victoria.ardiles@hospitalitaliano.org.ar

D. A. Biagiola
HPB Surgery and Liver Transplant Unit, Sanatorio Parque, Rosario, Argentina

J. Pekolj et al. (eds.), *Fundamentals of Bile Duct Injuries*,
https://doi.org/10.1007/978-3-031-13383-1_8

In fact, several studies have demonstrated that early diagnosis is a factor that has a significant influence on the results of initial and posterior treatment.

The initial clinical manifestation of patients presenting BDI is very heterogeneous, and a BDI must be suspected in even subtle deviations of the normal postoperative course following a cholecystectomy until proven otherwise. A high level of suspicion permits early diagnosis and the implementation of measures that will limit the damage [8].

The natural evolution of undiagnosed and untreated BDI always leads to multi-organ failure and mortality, either due to the presence of biliary obstruction, cholangitis, and sepsis or due to the presence of a biliary fistula that causes an abdominal collection (which may later infect) or a coleperitoneum that may result in biliary peritonitis. When these symptoms are present, the consequences on the patient are greater and the diagnosis becomes more evident [9].

Clinical Assessment

Clinical manifestations will mainly depend on the mechanism of the BDI. Thus, we can distinguish those originated by the biliary leak as a consequence of a partial or a total section of the biliary tree, from those originated by a partial or total obstruction of the bile's regular passage toward the duodenum.

Moreover, other factors affecting the clinical picture are the following: the presence of a bile leak and its volume, if it is localized or disseminated into the entire abdominal cavity, presence or not of an associated infection, concomitant vascular injury, and the time of diagnosis, i.e., the time of evolution of the complications associated with the occurrence of the injury [10].

The initial symptoms of BID can be extremely inconsistent. Abdominal pain and abdominal distention are insensitive criteria for diagnosing the presence of bile in the peritoneal cavity and, for an unpredictable time period, will be missing in many patients. One of the world's largest publications on BDI describes that only 27% of patients with abdominal distension, 23% with abdominal defense, and 13% with peritoneal signs. Evaluation of the patient will confirm or direct the suspicion on a case-by-case basis. In any patient with a poor postoperative course, BDI should be suspected and diagnostic methods should be implemented to confirm or exclude it [6].

According to the *type of injury* and the time of its evolution, we can identify different clinical situations:

Partial or Total Section of the Bile Duct

If the patient has an abdominal drain leading to the surgical site, bile leakage will be evident as it is localized and directed through the drain.

Bile leakage may present itself in three ways:

- *External bile leak:* This occurs in the early postoperative period, observing bile externalized through a drain. In such cases, we must suspect an aberrant unligated duct in the gallbladder bed (hepatocystic duct), the collapse of the cystic duct ligation or clip, or BID. Usually, in the first cases, the condition is limited to a biliary volume that disappears in a few days or may require endoscopic treatment with sphincterotomy and stent placement [11].
- *Biloma:* It is a localized bile collection as a result of a leak from the biliary tree. It might be asymptomatic, or most commonly have nonspecific digestive symptoms (dyspepsia, early satiety, or abdominal fullness). In patients with a larger biloma, it can cause inadequate gastric emptying, as well as abdominal pain localized in the right upper quadrant, which may be accompanied by anorexia, nausea, vomiting, and in some cases, homolateral shoulder pain [12].

If the diagnosis is delayed, this collection may become infected and transform into an abdominal abscess and should be suspected when the mentioned symptoms, septic manifestations are added. The diagnosis is confirmed with imaging studies.

- Choleperitoneum: It is a free biliary leakage inside the abdominal cavity. The clinical symptom is pain, usually diffuse, and of variable intensity. The choleperitoneum is usually well tolerated by the patient having little clinical repercussion to it. Abdominal distension, defense, and peritoneal signs are present in less than a third of patients. However, if this situation is maintained, the process will progressively evolve and may become infected, leading to biliary peritonitis [13].

This event will cause a greater impact on the patient's general condition with progressive deterioration and obvious septic signs. In some cases, associated jaundice may appear, which will suggest bile absorption by the peritoneum, sepsis, the addition of another injury that conditions a biliary obstruction, or a combination of the above.

Total or Partial obstruction of the Bile Flow

Jaundice is often accompanied by choluria (presence of bile pigments in urine) and acholia (lack of bile pigments in the stools). Bloodwork reveals cholestasis, characterized by elevated alkaline phosphatase (ALP) and hyperbilirubinemia (direct predominance). A progressively worsen cholestasis indicates a total obstruction. If associated with febrile syndrome, the patient may have acute cholangitis, which is a biliary emergency that needs to be treated urgently since it can rapidly progress to sepsis, shock, and multi-organ failure [14].

Endobiliary hypertension can easily translocate germs into the bloodstream, therefore cultures, broad-spectrum antibiotics covering Gram-negative germs and prompt biliary decompression is key [15].

Chronic obstruction of the biliary tree may also produce a progressive deterioration of liver function as irreversible consequences on the liver parenchyma, starting with fibrosis, portal hypertension, and culminating in secondary biliary cirrhosis (SBC) if left insufficiently treated. These changes are the result of unsuccessful secondary and tertiary prevention, i.e., failure to implement early diagnosis and different effective treatments [16, 17].

Complementary Studies

Numerous studies are available for the diagnosis and workup of a BDI. Most of them have been described in their respective section of this book. However, we think it is useful to review the most important ones and their application from a surgical perspective.

- Bloodwork: In cases of BDI with associated infection (cholangitis, abscesses, and peritonitis), the complete blood count might demonstrate an elevated white cell count with neutrophilia.

In cases of partial or total sections of the bile duct with external bile leak, the liver function tests (LFTs) should probably be normal.

In cases of minimal obstruction, only a modest increase in ALP and Gamma-Glutamyl Transpeptidase (GGT) will be observed with normal bilirubin values. Although in more severe obstruction, an increase in direct bilirubin and ALP will occur.

Transaminases, Alanine Aminotransferase (ALT), and Aspartate Aminotransferase (AST) will be elevated when there is repercussion in liver function due to cytolysis secondary to necrosis with or without coagulation disorders and other markers of liver function (International Normalized Ratio, Prothrombin time, Fibrinogen) usually occurring in cases with associated vascular disorders [4].

Multi-organ failure is accompanied by changes in renal function, metabolic acidosis, coagulopathy, and cytopenia, indicating the severity of the condition.

- IOC: When the anatomy is unclear in the context of acute or chronic inflammatory processes, the IOC can help to clear intraoperative uncertainties, enlightening our decision-making and preventing a BDI. Moreover, when a BDI occurred, and a bile leak is observed, IOC would facilitate its intraoperative diagnosis and extension, prevent its progression and eventually clear the way for a repair within the primary surgery. However, it should be considered that normal IOC may not exclude BID, since it still can be produced after the IOC [18–20].
- Ultrasonography (US): The US has numerous advantages. It is safe, low-cost, widely available, reliable, and thus, the first choice for biliary disease. It can detect:
  - Biliary dilatation: In patients with significant obstruction and several days of evolution, the bile duct may show a dominant intrahepatic dilatation. If the obstruction is partial, of recent evolution, or if there is an associated with an

  external bile leak, the bile duct will probably look normal since it has not been obstructed sufficiently to dilate.
  - Fluid collections: The most frequent sites are both subphrenic spaces, Morrison's fossa and pelvis that could require immediate resolution.
  - Liver parenchyma assessment: Looking for possible abscesses, hematomas, areas of ischemia, or doppler assessment to infer an associated vascular injury [21].

- CT scan: It can also detect bilomas and fluid collections in more deep locations, especially in obese patients. It also has the potential to be a guiding method for percutaneous treatment of intra-abdominal collections requiring evacuation and drainage. Early arterial phases (CT-angiography) have a high yield detecting ipsilateral arterial and/or portal injury, total hepatic pedicle injury, or associated pseudoaneurysm [22] (See Chap. 9).
- MRI / MRCP: The great advantage is that could provide a three-dimensional reconstruction of the biliary tree similarly to that achieved with PTC. With the advent of liver-specific contrasts, detection of uncertain bile leaks/bilomas has increased significantly as well. It is also a great tool to determine the status of the liver parenchyma and associated complications [23–25]. (See Chap. 9).
- Conventional Angiography: It is not routinely performed in the workup of a BID, although it is reasonable to do it when an associated vascular injury is uncertain (See Chap. 10).

There are specific circumstances we believe is key to including an angiographic assessment:

1. When there is a clear history of an arterial accident during surgery, which could have led to conversion, or to blind hemostatic salvage measures.
2. If complementary studies show images compatible with an ischemic sector of the liver.
3. When a patient is referred for medicolegal reasons the presence of an associated vascular lesion must always be confirmed.
4. When a previous repair has failed (stricture), in this case, there is more than a 50% probability that an associated vascular injury exists [26, 27].

- ERCP: provides a great possibility for biliary mapping through a technique called "Balloon Occlusion Cholangiogram" consisting of introducing a balloon in the distal CBD which permits a reasonable opacification of the biliary tree. Consequently, has a great potential to detect bile leaks caused by disruptions in the biliary tree and also facilitates deploying stents for their treatment. However, the limitations of the ERCP include a complete, and/or high (confluential) stenosis, since reaching the post stenosis biliary tree could be extremely difficult from below.

The disadvantage of the ERCP is still an invasive procedure requiring sedation and has complications, mainly related to the sphincterotomy, like acute pancreatitis, bleeding, and bowel perforation [28, 29] (See Chap. 13 Role of endoscopic procedures in the management of BDI).

- Percutaneous Transhepatic Cholangiography (PTC): This is used in the event of suspecting a BDI that compromises biliary confluence (high strictures), with upstream dilatation of the biliary tree and in which ERCP could not circumvent. It has the disadvantage of being an invasive procedure that can have complications related to liver puncture, radiation exposure, chances of reproducing cholangitis after contrast injection, and the need for a skilled interventional radiologist. Although its great advantage is that after the stenosis has been diagnosed, a Percutaneous Biliary Drainage (PBD) can be inserted to decompress the biliary tree [30].
- Sinusography: This is also a simple, low-cost study that can provide extremely valuable information on the mapping of the biliary tree. The only essential condition for this study is a reasonable time to establish a fistulous route through which the contrast can be injected (usually be at least 7 days). Antimicrobial prophylaxis should be indicated if the patient is not infected to avoid the possibility of reproducing acute cholangitis) [31] (See Chap. 12).

Conclusions

Secondary prevention of a BDI relies on early diagnosis (intraoperative or early postoperative) in order to limit the extent of the damage. The effectiveness of long-term treatment is influenced by the time of diagnosis. Therefore, in the presence of a torpid postoperative period from a gallbladder surgery which, normally is uneventful, a high suspicion of a BDI must be considered and aggressively ruled out.

References

1. Buddingh KT, Nieuwenhuijs VB, van Buuren L, Hulscher JBF, de Jong JS, van Dam GM. Intraoperative assessment of biliary anatomy for prevention of bile duct injury: a review of current and future patient safety interventions. Surg Endosc. 2011;25:2449–61.
2. Wu J-S, Peng C, Mao X-H, Lv P. Bile duct injuries associated with laparoscopic and open cholecystectomy: sixteen-year experience. World J Gastroenterol. 2007;13:2374–8.
3. Booij KAC, de Reuver PR, van Dieren S, van Delden OM, Rauws EA, Busch OR, van Gulik TM, Gouma DJ. Long-term impact of bile duct injury on morbidity, mortality, quality of life, and work related limitations. Ann Surg. 2018;268:143–50.
4. de' Angelis N, Catena F, Memeo R, et al. 2020 WSES guidelines for the detection and management of bile duct injury during cholecystectomy. World J Emerg Surg. 2021;16:30.
5. Moore DE, Feurer ID, Holzman MD, Wudel LJ, Strickland C, Gorden DL, Chari R, Wright JK, Pinson CW. Long-term detrimental effect of bile duct injury on health-related quality of life. Arch Surg. 2004;139:476–81. discussion 481–2
6. Jabłońska B, Lampe P. Iatrogenic bile duct injuries: etiology, diagnosis and management. World J Gastroenterol. 2009;15:4097–104.
7. Fong ZV, Pitt HA, Strasberg SM, Loehrer AP, Sicklick JK, Talamini MA, Lillemoe KD, Chang DC, California Cholecystectomy Group. Diminished survival in patients with bile leak and ductal injury: management strategy and outcomes. J Am Coll Surg. 2018;226:568–576.e1.

8. Archer SB, Brown DW, Smith CD, Branum GD, Hunter JG. Bile duct injury during laparoscopic cholecystectomy: results of a national survey. Ann Surg. 2001;234(549–58):discussion 558–9.
9. De Santibáñes E, Ardiles V, Pekolj J. Complex bile duct injuries: management HPB. 2008;10:4–12.
10. McMahon AJ, Fullarton G, Baxter JN, O'Dwyer PJ. Bile duct injury and bile leakage in laparoscopic cholecystectomy. Br J Surg. 1995;82:307–13.
11. Christoforidis E, Vasiliadis K, Goulimaris I, Tsalis K, Kanellos I, Papachilea T, Tsorlini E, Betsis D. A single center experience in minimally invasive treatment of postcholecystectomy bile leak, complicated with biloma formation. J Surg Res. 2007;141:171–5.
12. Bauer TW, Morris JB, Lowenstein A, Wolferth C, Rosato FE, Rosato EF. The consequences of a major bile duct injury during laparoscopic cholecystectomy. J Gastrointest Surg. 1998;2:61–6.
13. Walker AT, Shapiro AW, Brooks DC, Braver JM, Tumeh SS. Bile duct disruption and biloma after laparoscopic cholecystectomy: imaging evaluation. AJR Am J Roentgenol. 1992;158:785–9.
14. Takada T, Strasberg SM, Solomkin JS, et al. TG13: updated Tokyo guidelines for the management of acute cholangitis and cholecystitis. J Hepatobiliary Pancreat Sci. 2013;20:1–7.
15. Mohan R, Goh SWL, Tan GW, Tan YP, Junnarkar SP, Huey CWT, Low JK, Shelat VG. Validation of Tokyo guidelines 2007 and Tokyo guidelines 2013/2018 criteria for acute cholangitis and predictors of in-hospital mortality. Visceral Medicine. 2021;37:434–42.
16. Negi SS, Sakhuja P, Malhotra V, Chaudhary A. Factors predicting advanced hepatic fibrosis in patients with postcholecystectomy bile duct strictures. Arch Surg. 2004;139:299–303.
17. Desantibanes E, Pekolj J, Mccormack L, Nefa J, Acuna J, Mattera J, Gadano A, Sivori J, Ciardullo M. 180Liver transplantation for intraoperative biliary tree injuries. Liver Transpl. 2000;6:C45.
18. Rystedt JML, Wiss J, Adolfsson J, Enochsson L, Hallerbäck B, Johansson P, Jönsson C, Leander P, Österberg J, Montgomery A. Routine versus selective intraoperative cholangiography during cholecystectomy: systematic review, meta-analysis and health economic model analysis of iatrogenic bile duct injury. BJS Open. 2021; https://doi.org/10.1093/bjsopen/zraa032.
19. Alvarez FA, de Santibañes M, Palavecino M, Sánchez Clariá R, Mazza O, Arbues G, de Santibañes E, Pekolj J. Impact of routine intraoperative cholangiography during laparoscopic cholecystectomy on bile duct injury. Br J Surg. 2014;101:677–84.
20. Pekolj J, Alvarez FA, Palavecino M, Sánchez Clariá R, Mazza O, de Santibañes E. Intraoperative management and repair of bile duct injuries sustained during 10,123 laparoscopic cholecystectomies in a high-volume referral center. J Am Coll Surg. 2013;216:894–901.
21. Melamud K, LeBedis CA, Anderson SW, Soto JA. Biliary imaging: multimodality approach to imaging of biliary injuries and their complications. Radiographics. 2014;34:613–23.
22. Yeh BM, Liu PS, Soto JA, Corvera CA, Hussain HK. MR imaging and CT of the biliary tract. Radiographics. 2009;29:1669–88.
23. Hyodo T, Kumano S, Kushihata F, Okada M, Hirata M, Tsuda T, Takada Y, Mochizuki T, Murakami T. CT and MR cholangiography: advantages and pitfalls in perioperative evaluation of biliary tree. Br J Radiol. 2012;85:887–96.
24. Reddy S, Lopes Vendrami C, Mittal P, Borhani AA, Moreno CC, Miller FH. MRI evaluation of bile duct injuries and other post-cholecystectomy complications. Abdom Radiol (NY). 2021;46:3086–104.
25. Médart L, Coibion C, Deflandre J. Hepatobiliary-specific contrast agent in biliary leak. JBR-BTR. 2018;102:58.
26. Keleman AM, Imagawa DK, Findeiss L, et al. Associated vascular injury in patients with bile duct injury during cholecystectomy. Am Surg. 2011;77:1330–3.
27. Machado NO, Al-Zadjali A, Kakaria AK, Younus S, Rahim MA, Al-Sukaiti R. Hepatic or cystic artery Pseudoaneurysms following a laparoscopic cholecystectomy: literature review of aetiopathogenesis, presentation, diagnosis and management. Sultan Qaboos Univ Med J. 2017;17:e135–46.

28. Nordin A, Halme L, Mäkisalo H, Isoniemi H, Höckerstedt K. Management and outcome of major bile duct injuries after laparoscopic cholecystectomy: from therapeutic endoscopy to liver transplantation. Liver Transpl. 2002;8:1036–43.
29. Shah JN. Endoscopic treatment of bile leaks: current standards and recent innovations. Gastrointest Endosc. 2007;65:1069–72.
30. Misra S, Melton GB, Geschwind JF, Venbrux AC, Cameron JL, Lillemoe KD. Percutaneous management of bile duct strictures and injuries associated with laparoscopic cholecystectomy: a decade of experience. J Am Coll Surg. 2004;198:218–26.
31. Thompson CM, Saad NE, Quazi RR, Darcy MD, Picus DD, Menias CO. Management of iatrogenic bile duct injuries: role of the interventional radiologist. Radiographics. 2013;33:117–34.

Chapter 9
Role of Imaging

Juan Carlos Spina and Ramiro Orta

Introduction

Imaging methods have a protagonistic role in Bile Duct Injuries (BDI) along with different circumstances:

- Preventively, the ultrasound (US) can alert the surgeon to anticipate a potential challenging case.
- Intraoperatively, the Intraoperative Cholangiogram (IOC) or the laparoscopic US can enlighten the anatomical uncertainties that predispose to BDIs playing a fundamental role in their prevention [1].
- If a BDI has been established, can be diagnosed at the time of surgery using IOC, or either in the early or late postoperative period using the US, Computed Tomography (CT) scan, Magnetic Resonance Imaging/Magnetic Resonance Cholangiopancreatography (MRI/MRCP) offer different diagnostic benefits depending on the time of presentation and the patient's clinical condition [2, 3].

Prevention

US is widely accepted as the method of choice for the *initial* study of the gallbladder and biliary tract. Its role in the risk stratification of complex biliary pathology is unquestionable.

J. C. Spina (✉)
Body Imaging, HBP Section, Hospital Italiano de Buenos Aires, Buenos Aires, Argentina
e-mail: juan.spina@hospitalitaliano.org.ar

R. Orta
Body Imaging, HBP Section, Sanatorio Parque, Rosario, Argentina

J. Pekolj et al. (eds.), *Fundamentals of Bile Duct Injuries*,
https://doi.org/10.1007/978-3-031-13383-1_9

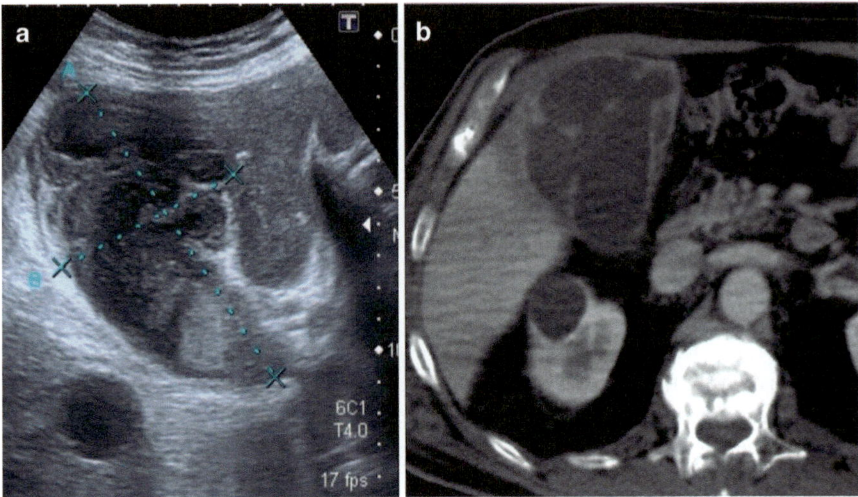

Fig. 9.1 Ultrasound (US) (**a**) shows an enlarged gallbladder with thick walls and heterogeneous contents. (**b**) Computed tomography (CT) scan confirms these findings and shows areas of wall disruption in favor of perivesicular abscesses

In this sense, acute cholecystitis (AC), exacerbated chronic cholecystitis (CC), and scleroatrophic gallbladders imply a higher risk of surgical treatment and can be easily detected by the routine US [4].

Those signs include a very thickened gallbladder wall (greater than 10 mm), cholelithiasis impacted in the infundibulum, and the presence of abscess or perivesicular plastron [5], Fig. 9.1.

A collapsed or fluidless gallbladder with or without parietal calcifications is usually related to scleroatrophic changes. The presence of dilatation of intrahepatic bile ducts, associated with dilatation of the proximal sector of the extrahepatic ducts should suggest Mirizzi syndrome. In addition, dilatation of the distal extrahepatic ducts may be associated with choledochal lithiasis, not always visible in US.

Abdominal CT scan and MRI are not first-line methods for the study of gallbladder pathology and are usually reserved for acute or chronic cholecystitis with extensive local involvement or to rule out gallbladder cancer [6].

MRCP is particularly useful for confirmation of Mirizzi's syndrome and for choledochal lithiasis not visible by US, as well as allowing a correct evaluation of the biliary anatomy in order to detect variants with significant implications for surgery [7, 8] Fig. 9.2.

Whether or not IOC should be used systematically and selectively is still a matter of debate. What has been demonstrated is that IOC helps to detect an early injury, preventing the progression of damage and thus further related complications [9] (See Chap. 7).

A multicenter study including 1381 patients assessed the routine use of laparoscopic US in gallbladder surgery. This study demonstrated that routine use of

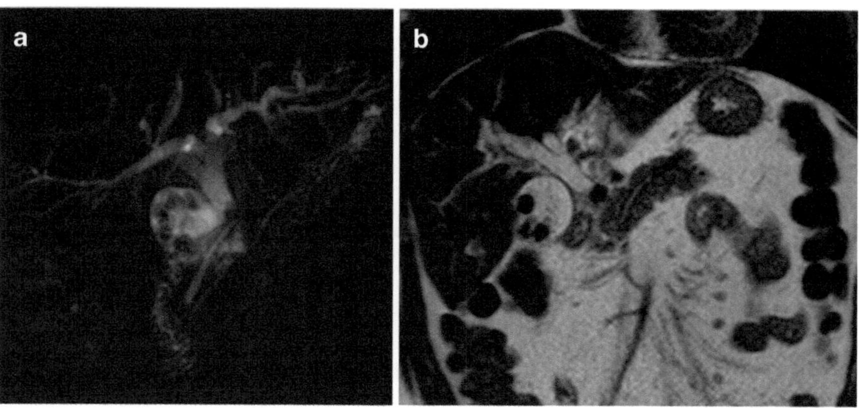

Fig. 9.2 (**a**) MRCP and (**b**) coronal T2WI sequence showing an image of a filling defect in the cystic duct which imprints on the common bile duct (CBD) with upstream dilatation, favoring a Mirizzi syndrome

laparoscopic US during LC has significantly improved its safety, compared to the previously reported BDI prevention rates (1 out of 200–400 LCs) [10]. The main issue is that laparoscopic US probes are often expensive and not widely available. Moreover, requires training and experience to achieve the best results.

Diagnosis of a BDI in the Early Postoperative Period

The most complex scenario is when the BDI occurred and was not recognized during the primary surgery.

In this situation, the patient is seen within the first week of the postoperative period with abdominal pain, peritonitis, sepsis, and overall poor general condition.

Any patient presenting like this after an elective cholecystectomy should be worked up, with a high suspicion of a BDI. The preferred initial studies are US and CT scan.

The presence of free peritoneal fluid, a perihepatic collection, or a fluid collection that lies adjacent to the CBD, with or without dilatation in the mentioned clinical context could represent indirect signs of a BDI, Fig. 9.3.

Should the BDI be confirmed, efforts at this stage should be directed to stabilize the patient and control the sepsis. The imaging is important to conduct therapies to address the acute disturbances the patient is facing, such as draining localized fluid collections or indicating abdominal washout in case of a choleperitoneum. More detailed studies should be deferred once the first objective (compensating and getting the patient out of the "danger zone") is achieved.

CT scan has some advantages over the US in delineating abdominal fluid collections as well as in their therapeutic planning their percutaneous drainage is necessary, Fig. 9.4.

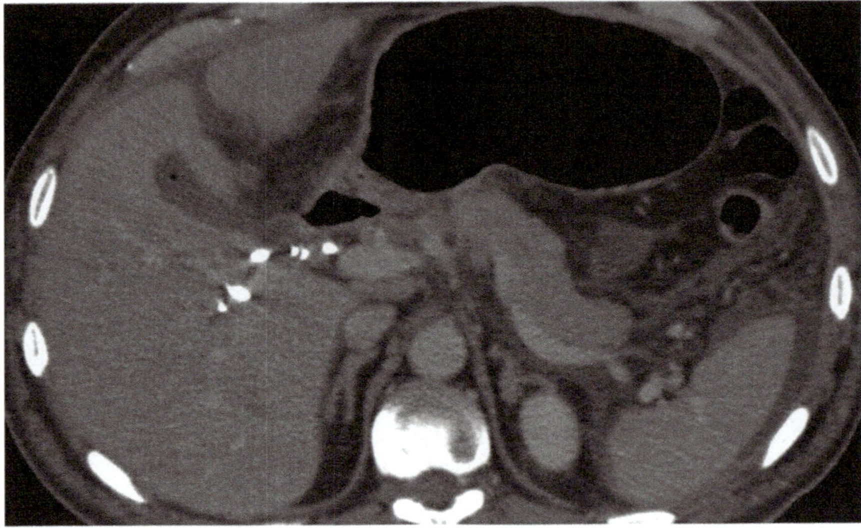

Fig. 9.3 CT scan with intravenous contrast of a patient in the postoperative period of a cholecystectomy. Free peritoneal fluid, perihepatic, perisplenic, and in the lesser sac can be appreciated. Note the numerous metallic clips in the gallbladder fossa, which are suggestive of complicated cholecystectomy

Fig. 9.4 Axial view of intravenous contrast-enhanced CT scan. Hydroaerial collection in the gallbladder bed (arrows) in a patient who underwent a laparoscopic cholecystectomy

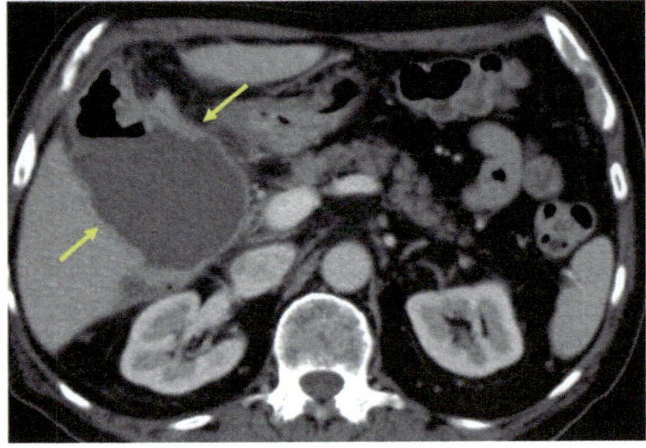

Diagnosis of a BDI in the Late Postoperative Period

BDIs that have gone unnoticed during the primary surgery and have not shown early symptoms, usually manifest later with fewer press symptoms.

These subacute manifestations of BDIs occur as a result of either partial or complete stenosis of secondary to metallic clips, thermal injuries causing progressive fibrosis or scarring or ischemia of the biliary tree. Symptoms are usually manifestations of cholestasis and include jaundice, pruritus, and cholangitis.

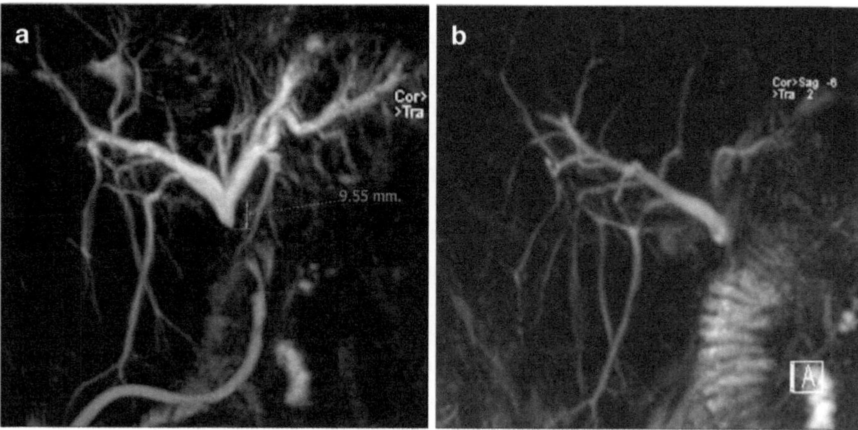

Fig. 9.5 MRCP showing a stenosis of the CBD secondary to BDI. (**a**) An interruption of the signal in the CBD with an indemnity of its proximal portion—*estimated at 9* mm—an upstream dilatation of the biliary tree can be appreciated. (**b**) MRCP after reconstruction using a Roux-en-Y Hepaticojejunostomy (**b**)

MRCP represents the method of choice for the evaluation of biliary anatomy at this stage. The presence of a sector of the biliary duct with a reduction in caliber or interruption of the signal allows the diagnosis of partial or complete stenosis, respectively. The localization of the extension of the stenosis can be determined with precision using this method, and the extent of the injury can be measured as well allowing precise surgical planning [7], Fig. 9.5.

Planning Surgical Reconstruction

Restoring the bilioenteric continuity and preventing cholestasis is the main priority once BDI's had been compensated in the acute phase.

At this point, the main role of imaging is to define as accurately as possible the type of BDI the patient has and whether or not it is accompanied by vascular injury.

Is key to knowing if there's biliary dilatation, any repercussion in the liver parenchyma, or if any other finding throughout the abdomen needs to be addressed as well.

All this information will play a fundamental role in the preparation for reconstructive surgery and will determine which is the best surgical approach.

Navigating the Uncertainties

In patients with a BDI, the diagnostic accuracy of conventional MRI/MRCP to detect a bile leak is about 70%. For the rest of the cases, or when there are some uncertainties about the location of the BDI (marked inflammation, collections, surgical clips, or drains either in the biliary tree or in the right upper quadrant), we can utilize other methods to better identify this [11].

Hepatobiliary Scintigraphy (HBS) is a widely available and economic method to detect the presence of bile leak, however, it lacks anatomical detail to aid in treatment planning [12].

Until a few years ago, this information was provided by Endoscopic Retrograde Cholangiopancreatography (ERCP) was the gold standard as it allows to identify directly and dynamically the presence of contrast extravasation outside the biliary tree at the site of the BDI and provides the window for therapeutic stent placements if necessary.

However, does not provide information about the status of the biliary duct proximal to the site of the BDI when the section is complete. In addition, as an invasive procedure is not exempt from complications (acute pancreatitis, infection, etc.) See Chap. 13.

Hepato-specific contrast Gadoxetic Disodium Acid (Gd-EOB-DTPA, Primovist), is a type of Gadolinium that has the characteristic of a rapid distribution in the bloodstream and a dual elimination pathway (50% renal and 50% biliar), combining the characteristic of conventional extracellular contrast agent with those hepato-specific.

Due to its chemical composition, it is taken up by the hepatocyte and then eliminated via the biliary system. It is worth mentioning that the uptake of hepatocyte-specific contrast is mediated by the same membrane transporter as bilirubin. Therefore, the lack of opacification of the biliary tree 20–30 mins after contrast administration may suggest biliary obstruction or poor liver function [13].

Its main indication classically lay in the detection and distinction of focal hepatic injuries (focal nodular hyperplasia vs. adenomas; determination of the number of hepatic metastases or characterization of nodules in cirrhotic patients) [14].

Recently, MRI with hepato-specific agents has been shown to provide dynamic and functional information on the biliary excretion and indirectly on liver function as well, similar to HBS.

Their role in the management of BDI lies in the fact that has the capacity of performing accurate cholangiograms since demonstrate the biliary anatomy in a similar way to an MRCP, although with direct excreted contrast [13], Fig. 9.6.

It also allows Imaging methods: detection of active bile leak at the site of the BDI by direct visualization of the passage of contrast into the perihepatic or peribiliary fluid collections. This finding is represented by the presence of hyperintense signals in T1 sequences within these collections in images obtained in the hepatobiliary phase (20–60 mins). This then allows a correct noninvasive differential diagnoses between a BDI biloma and other possible etiologies of liquid collections near the surgical site (abscess, hematoma, cysts) [15].

Kantarci et al. demonstrated that the combination of conventional MRI + MRI cholangiography with hepato-specific contrast significantly increases the detection of BDI with associated bile leak [16].

In their series, they demonstrated that the identification of the BDI site using conventional MRCP was Imaging methods: obtained in 50% of patients but

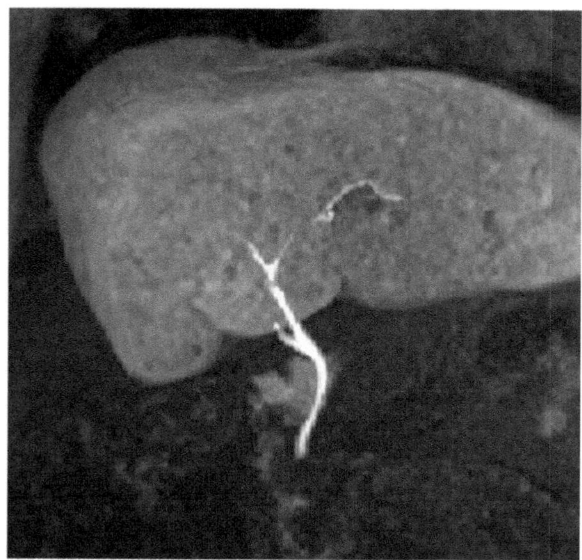

Fig. 9.6 MRCP with hepato-specific contrast. Both the intrahepatic and the extrahepatic biliary tree does not show signs of dilatation. Note the cystic duct stump post-cholecystectomy

increased to a sensitivity of 81.2% and a specificity of 100% when combined with MRI with hepatocyte-specific agents.

In patients with a late manifestation of biliary stenosis, MRCP with hepato-specific agents can provide additional information about the degree of stenosis (partial or complete) based on the demonstration of contrast in the distal common bile duct below the site of stenosis as well [17].

Vascular Evaluation

The presence of a concomitant vascular injury has a variable incidence that depends on the type of BDI (See Chap. 6). However, the most frequent is an associated injury to the right hepatic artery (RHA) given its close relationship with the CBD (it runs posterior to the CBD in 71.6% and anterior in 8.3%) [18].

The development of an anastomotic network from the left hepatic artery (LHA) in general through the hilar plexus can supply sufficiently the irrigation of the right biliary tree. However, when the damage includes the portal vein (PV) as well, the risk of hepatic and biliary necrosis increases significantly [19].

A routine examination of the hepatic vasculature is recommended in every BDI, although it is fundamental to have it worked up when planning a reconstructive surgery.

The advent of CT scan with multiplanar and three-dimensional reconstructions has made significant progress in the assessment of vascular anatomy of the liver. CT Angiography is now an adequate tool for the assessment of associated vascular lesions, detecting direct signs of associated vascular injury such as the presence of

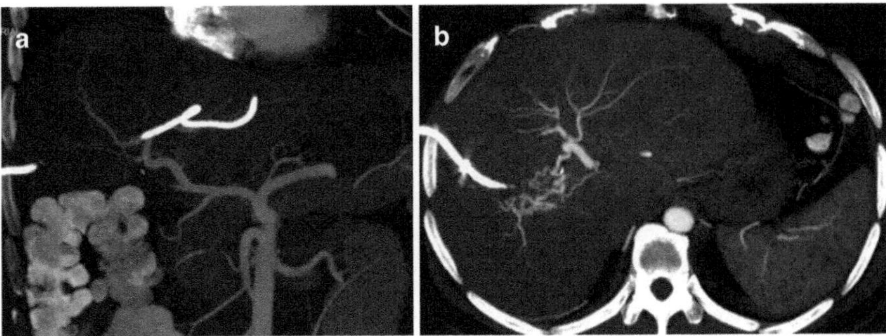

Fig. 9.7 MIP reconstructions from a CT angiography of a patient with BDI. (**a**) The coronal section shows amputation of the right hepatic artery. (**b**) The axial section shows the collateralization through an anastomotic network provided by the left hepatic artery

thinning, irregularity, or amputation of an artery, as well as the formation of pseudoaneurysms [20, 21] (See Chap. 11).

Indirect signs of vascular injury include areas of hepatic parenchymal infarction and necrosis, abscesses, lobar atrophy, and failure of attempted repair of a bilioenteric anastomosis, Fig. 9.7.

Conclusions

Imaging has a decisive role in every stage of a BDI, from prevention to ultimate management.

Preoperative US and MRI can warn of the likelihood of difficult cholecystectomy, while the use of IOC contributes to the early diagnosis of the lesion injury and avoids further damage if the intraoperative imaging is interpreted correctly.

If the BDI happened to occur, the abdominal US and CT scan represent the first-line methods addressing the patient's immediate needs (sepsis, fluid collections, peritonitis, perforation, etc.).

MRI/MRCP and the use of hepato-specific agents provide a correct evaluation of the biliary anatomy with the detection of possible bile leaks.

Finally, the use of CT angiography allows a precise characterization of the associated vascular injuries, decisive for planning the resolution of the BDI.

References

1. Alvarez FA, de Santibañes M, Palavecino M, Sánchez Clariá R, Mazza O, Arbues G, de Santibañes E, Pekolj J. Impact of routine intraoperative cholangiography during laparoscopic cholecystectomy on bile duct injury. Br J Surg. 2014;101:677–84.
2. Melamud K, LeBedis CA, Anderson SW, Soto JA. Biliary imaging: multimodality approach to imaging of biliary injuries and their complications. Radiographics. 2014;34:613–23.

3. Yeh BM, Liu PS, Soto JA, Corvera CA, Hussain HK. MR imaging and CT of the biliary tract. Radiographics. 2009;29:1669–88.
4. Elshaer M, Gravante G, Thomas K, Sorge R, Al-Hamali S, Ebdewi H. Subtotal cholecystectomy for "difficult gallbladders": systematic review and meta-analysis. JAMA Surg. 2015;150:159–68.
5. de' Angelis N, Catena F, Memeo R, et al. 2020 WSES guidelines for the detection and management of bile duct injury during cholecystectomy. World J Emerg Surg. 2021;16:30.
6. Hyodo T, Kumano S, Kushihata F, Okada M, Hirata M, Tsuda T, Takada Y, Mochizuki T, Murakami T. CT and MR cholangiography: advantages and pitfalls in the perioperative evaluation of the biliary tree. Br J Radiol. 2012;85:887–96.
7. Reddy S, Lopes Vendrami C, Mittal P, Borhani AA, Moreno CC, Miller FH. MRI evaluation of bile duct injuries and other post-cholecystectomy complications. Abdom Radiol (NY). 2021;46:3086–104.
8. Md LM. The Mirizzi syndrome –major cause for biliary duct injury during laparoscopic cholecystectomy. Biomed J Sci Tech Res. 2017;1 https://doi.org/10.26717/bjstr.2017.01.000308.
9. Rystedt JML, Wiss J, Adolfsson J, Enochsson L, Hallerbäck B, Johansson P, Jönsson C, Leander P, Österberg J, Montgomery A. Routine versus selective intraoperative cholangiography during cholecystectomy: systematic review, meta-analysis and health economic model analysis of iatrogenic bile duct injury. BJS Open. 2021;5 https://doi.org/10.1093/bjsopen/zraa032.
10. Machi J, Johnson JO, Deziel DJ, Soper NJ, Berber E, Siperstein A, Hata M, Patel A, Singh K, Arregui ME. The routine use of laparoscopic ultrasound decreases bile duct injury: a multicenter study. Surg Endosc. 2009;23:384–8.
11. Aduna M, Larena JA, Martín D, Martínez-Guereñu B, Aguirre I, Astigarraga E. Bile duct leaks after laparoscopic cholecystectomy: value of contrast-enhanced MRCP. Abdom Imaging. 2005;30:480–7.
12. Sharma P, Kumar R, Das KJ, Singh H, Pal S, Parshad R, Bal C, Bandopadhyaya GP, Malhotra A. Detection and localization of post-operative and post-traumatic bile leak: hybrid SPECT-CT with 99mTc-Mebrofenin. Abdom Imaging. 2012;37:803–11.
13. Gupta RT, Brady CM, Lotz J, Boll DT, Merkle EM. Dynamic MR imaging of the biliary system using hepatocyte-specific contrast agents. AJR Am J Roentgenol. 2010;195:405–13.
14. Grazioli L, Olivetti L, Mazza G, Bondioni MP. MR imaging of hepatocellular adenomas and differential diagnosis dilemma. Int J Hepatol. 2013;2013:374170.
15. Médart L, Coibion C, Deflandre J. Hepatobiliary-specific contrast agent in biliary leak. JBR-BTR. 2018;102:58.
16. Kantarcı M, Pirimoglu B, Karabulut N, Bayraktutan U, Ogul H, Ozturk G, Aydinli B, Kizrak Y, Eren S, Yilmaz S. Non-invasive detection of biliary leaks using Gd-EOB-DTPA-enhanced MR cholangiography: comparison with T2-weighted MR cholangiography. Eur Radiol. 2013;23:2713–22.
17. Lee NK, Kim S, Lee JW, Lee SH, Kang DH, Kim GH, Seo HI. Biliary MR imaging with Gd-EOB-DTPA and its clinical applications. Radiographics. 2009;29:1707–24.
18. Dandekar U, Dandekar K, Chavan S. Right hepatic artery: a cadaver investigation and its clinical significance. Anat Res Int. 2015;2015:412595.
19. Buell JF, Cronin DC, Funaki B, Koffron A, Yoshida A, Lo A, Leef J, Millis JM. Devastating and fatal complications associated with combined vascular and bile duct injuries during cholecystectomy. Arch Surg. 2002;137:703–8. discussion 708–10
20. Madanur MA, Battula N, Sethi H, Deshpande R, Heaton N, Rela M. Pseudoaneurysm following laparoscopic cholecystectomy. Hepatobiliary Pancreat Dis Int. 2007;6:294–8.
21. Machado NO, Al-Zadjali A, Kakaria AK, Younus S, Rahim MA, Al-Sukaiti R. Hepatic or cystic artery Pseudoaneurysms following a laparoscopic cholecystectomy: literature review of aetiopathogenesis, presentation, diagnosis and management. Sultan Qaboos Univ Med J. 2017;17:e135–46.

Chapter 10
Assessment of Vascular Structures in BDI's

David Alberto Biagiola and Martín de Santibañes

Introduction

In this section, we will analyze the study of the vascular tree in the setting of a Bile Duct Injury (BDI) and the importance of ruling out any associated vascular injury (AVI) when they occur. This factor is fundamental to not only determine the most appropriate reparative strategy but also would play a preponderant role in the ultimate outcome [1].

In consequence, a comprenhensive workuo to rule out any AVI, beyond the biliary compromise, is mandatory [2].

Clinical Manifestation of AVI

The incidence of AVI varies between 27% and 61%. Koffron et al. report that in more than 60% of failed attempts of surgical repair of BDI, an AVI was further demonstrated [3].

As a rule of thumb, the more proximal the biliary injury, the more frequently an AVI is found.

D. A. Biagiola
HPB Surgery and Liver Transplant Unit, Sanatorio Parque, Rosario, Argentina

M. de Santibañes (✉)
HPB Surgery and Liver Transplant Unit, Hospital Italiano de Buenos Aires, Buenos Aires, Argentina
e-mail: martin.desantibanes@hospitalitaliano.org.ar

J. Pekolj et al. (eds.), *Fundamentals of Bile Duct Injuries*, https://doi.org/10.1007/978-3-031-13383-1_10

Occasionally, conventional imaging does not demonstrate an obvious associated vascular injury, although we can suspect one based on indirect signs such as hepatic ischemia or necrosis, lobar atrophy, cirrhosis, portal hypertension, or failure of the first attempt of surgical repair with a hepaticojejunostomy (HJ) [4].

Parenchymal atrophy, which is usually secondary to hepatic ischemia, may have an asymptomatic course, especially when it is limited to one lobe of the liver. However, a lack of compensation from the healthy side will result in liver necrosis with parenchymal abscesses and eventually liver failure [5, 6]. The liver parenchyma can have atrophy as a result of biliary stenosis and successive episodes of cholangitis [7].

Hemobilia is another manifestation related to communication between vascular structures and the biliary duct. It is often related to a pseudoaneurysm of the hepatic artery or cystic artery. It represents a relatively rare cause of upper gastrointestinal hemorrhage, but with high mortality [8].

The pathogenesis of a *pseudoaneurysm* is unclear, but it is suspected that direct injury to the vessel wall is caused by diverse factors like chronic bile leak, infection, erosion from a metal clip or direct thermal injury to the vessel. Also, long standing drains, or manipulation of percutaneous drains and wires could play a role in their formation [9, 10].

Vascular Compensatory System

The most commonly affected vascular structure in a BDI is the right hepatic artery (RHA) due to its anatomical relationship to common bile duct (CBD). The RHA runs posterior to the CBD in 71.6% and anterior in 8.3% of the cases [11].

Less frequently, the right branch of the portal vein (PV) can suffer an AVI or the main trunk of both artery and vein. This mixed injury (arterial and venous) can coexist and should always be suspected [12].

Often an AVI might not have clinical consequences whatsoever. It will depend on the level of the injury, and if, accordingly, the collateralization at the level of the hilar plexus remains preserved. This natural compensatory system can partially or totally provide irrigation to the area of the liver supplied by the injured vessel [2].

This complex vascular network system is represented by collateralization that frequently comes from:

- Left hepatic artery (LHA).
- Superior mesenteric artery (SMA) via the gastroduodenal artery (GDA), pancreaticoduodenals (PDs), retroduodenal and retroportal arteries.
- Epi-choledochal arterial plexus.
- Marginal arteries of the CBD (located at hours 9 and 3).
- Transverse hilar marginal artery.

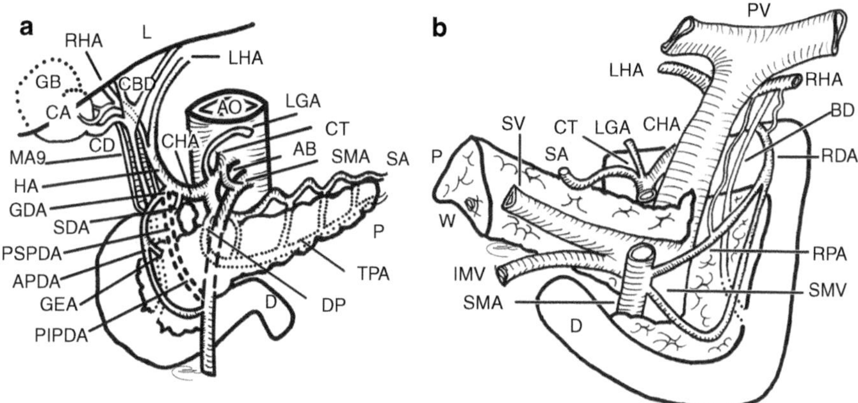

Fig. 10.1 Blood supply of the biliary tree. (**a**) The bile ducts are vascularized by branches of the *Cystic Artery (CA)* anteriorly and branches of the *Pancreaticoduodenal Artery (PDA)* posteriorly. The vascularization of the upper part comes from the CA and the lower part from the *Hepatic Artery (HA), Gastroduodenal Artery (GDA), or Supraduodenal arteries (SDA)*. (**b**) The pericholedochal arterial plexus derive from the posterior superior and retroduodenal PDAs. References L: Liver; GB: Gallbladder; CBD: Common Bile Duct; P: Pancreas; D: Duodenum; CHA: Common Hepatic Artery; RHA: Right Hepatic Artery; LHA: Left Hepatic Artery; CD: Cystic Duct; Ao: Aorta; CT: Celiac Trunk; SMA: Superior Mesenteric Artery; LGA: Left Gastric Artery; SA: Splenic Artery; PSPDA: Posterior Superior Pancreaticoduodenal Artery; APDA: Anterior Pancreaticoduodenal Artery; PIPDA: Posterior Inferior Pancreaticoduodenal Artery. MA9: Marginal Artery hour 9; GDA: Gastroduodenal Artery; GEA: Gastroepiploic Artery; DP: Dorsal Pancreatic Artery; TPA: Transverse Pancreatic Artery; RPA: Retroportal Artery; RDA: Retroduodenal Artery; PV: Portal Vein; SV: Splenic Vein; SMV: Superior Mesenteric Vein; IMV: Inferior Mesenteric Vein

- Transverse hilar plexus.
- Replaced (aberrant) or accessory hepatic arteries.
- Arc of Buhler (AOB): occasionally persistent anastomosis between the 10th and 13th ventral segmental arteries, that results in communication between the celiac trunk and SMA. This arch is independent of both the dorsal pancreatic artery and GDA [13–15] (Figs. 10.1, 10.2 and 10.3).

In general, a high RHA injury triggers compensatory intrahepatic, longitudinal and transverse shunt systems without significantly affecting the hepatic perfusion [16] (Fig. 10.4).

Strasberg E1–E3 injuries lead to the longitudinal shunt of the marginals being obstructed at the level of the injury and would be compensated through the left to right transverse hilar shunt, causing the distal segment of the vascular injury to the RHA to be perfused regardless [17] (Fig. 10.5a).

However, in Strasberg E4 injuries, as the biliary confluence is involved along with the AVI to the RHA, both the longitudinal shunt of the marginals and the

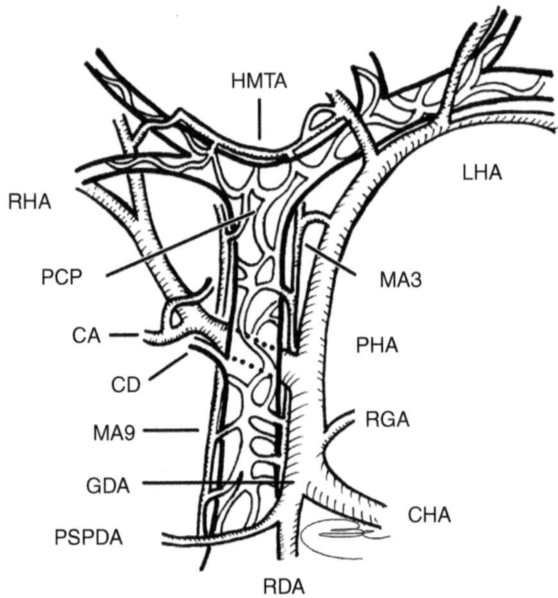

Fig. 10.2 Arterial plexus. The pericholedochal arterial plexus of the CBD originating from the PDAs, PSPDA, and RDA are pictured. The marginal arteries of hours 3 and 9 branching of the GDA and PPSPDA are observed. The marginal lines of the transverse hilum arise above the left hepatic artery. PDA: Pancreaticoduodenal Arteries; PSPDA: Posterior Superior Pancreaticoduodenal Artery; RDA: Retroduodenal Arteries; GDA: Gastroduodenal Artery; PSPDA: Posterior Superior Pancreaticoduodenal Arteries. CHA: Common Hepatic Artery; PHA: Proper Hepatic Artery; RHA: Right Hepatic Artery; LHA: Left Hepatic Artery; CD: Cystic Duct; RGA: Right Gastric Artery. HMTA: Hilar Marginal Transverse Arteries; PCP: Pericholedochal Plexus; PSPDA: Posterior Superior Pancreaticoduodenal Artery; MA3: marginal Artery hour 3; MA9: Marginal Artery hour 9

transverse hilar plexus will be compromised. Therefore, the right hemiliver will lack an arterial compensatory inflow circuit. As consequence, the right lobe of the liver will have a high risk of ischemia and intrahepatic ischemic cholangiopathy [18] (Fig. 10.5b).

It is also important that the presence of an arcuate ligament syndrome (ALS) can be completely asymptomatic, although gains relevance in the setting of a BDI with AVI. Its presence will naturally predispose to a relative reduction in the hepatic arterial inflow and thus compromise the LHA that would ideally compensate for a RHA injury [19, 20].

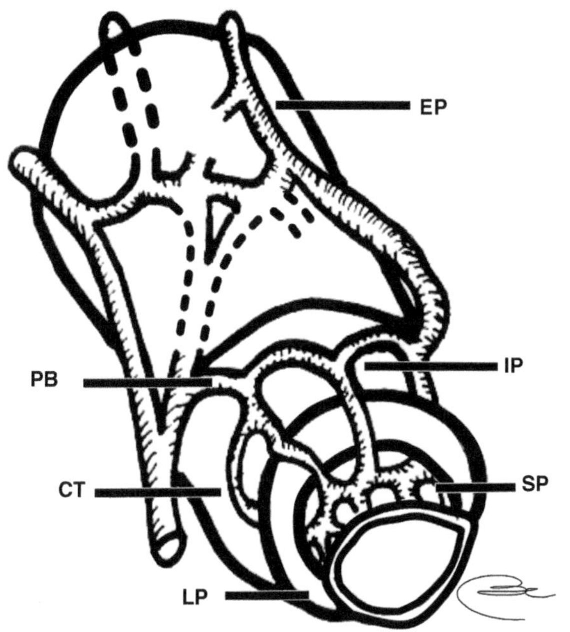

Fig. 10.3 Collateral Circulation. It is developed by two plexuses, the extrinsic formed by the Epi-coledocholedochal arterial plexus with perforating branches and the intrinsic formed by the intramural and subepithelial plexus. EP: Extrinsic Plexus; IP: Intramural Plexus; SP: Subepithelial Plexus; PB: Perforating branch; CT: Connective Tissue; LP: Lamina Propria

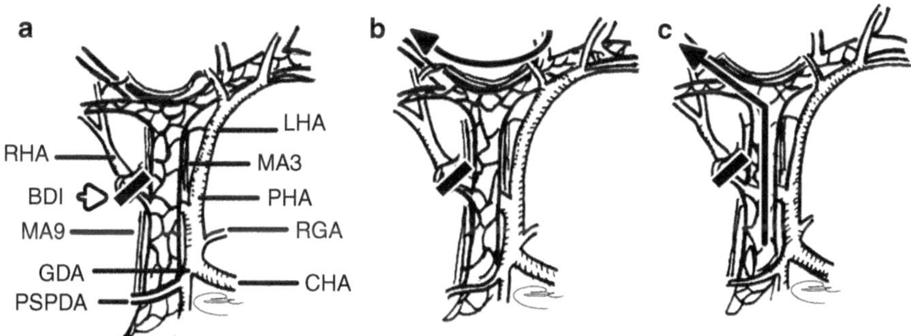

Fig. 10.4 Hepatic blood flow in RHA injury without BDI. (**a**) *RHA* occlusion (white arrowhead), with the restored flow by collateral arterial shunts. (**b**) Hilar transverse marginal arterial shunt. (**c**) Epicholedochal plexus longitudinal arterial shunt. BDI: Bile Duct Injury; CHA: Common Hepatic Artery; PHA: Proper Hepatic Artery; RHA: Right Hepatic Artery; LHA: Left Hepatic Artery; RGA: Right Gastric Artery. PSPDA: Posterior Superior Pancreaticoduodenal Artery; MA3: marginal Artery hour 3; MA9: Marginal Artery hour 9; GDA: Gastroduodenal Artery

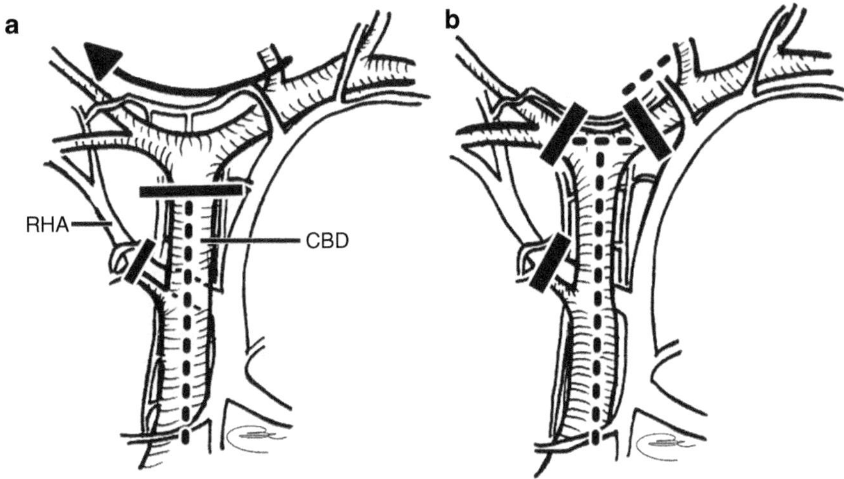

Fig. 10.5 The injury affects the RHA and the CBD at different levels. (**a**) Strasberg E1–3 injuries allow irrigation of the right liver through the transverse hilar shunt (black arrow) but compromise the longitudinal shunt (dotted line). (**b**) Strasberg E4 injuries induce greater ischemia due to obstruction of both transverse and longitudinal shunts (dotted line). RHA: Right Hepatic Artery; CBD: Common Bile Duct

Diagnosis

CT scan and Magnetic Resonance Imaging (MRI) are routine non-invasive imaging studies in the assessment of BID and its associated complications such as abdominal collection, liver abscess, and lobar atrophy. At the same time, the development of CT-angiography protocols facilitated by modern equipment and processing software has made it possible to acquire non-invasively very precise hepatic vascular imaging. Thanks to the three-dimensional reconstructions pseudoaneurysms are easier to diagnose as well [21].

Moreover, within a sagittal view, the CT scan can accurately reveal the existence of ALS. As we mentioned before, it might predispose to a relative reduction in the hepatic arterial inflow and could indicate to associate an ALS release procedure during the reconstructive surgery for the BDI [22].

However, there are circumstances in which *hepatic angiography* plays a crucial role. Despite being an invasive study, its indication is given when the diagnosis of AVI is uncertain or to diagnose and eventually treat a *pseudoaneurysm* [23].

The importance of diagnosing an AVI lies in establishing the best surgical strategy for a definitive resolution of the BDI, but it is also important to have concrete documentation of the situation for medico-legal reasons (Figs. 10.6 and 10.7).

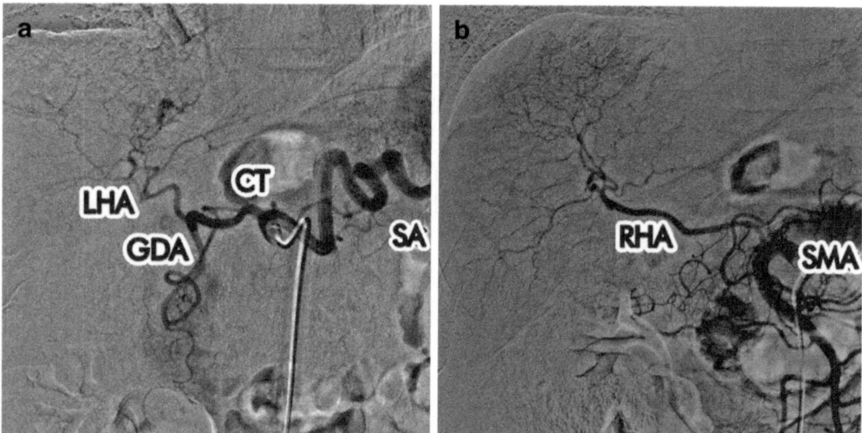

Fig. 10.6 Digital angiography case I. (**a**) The LHA branches of the CT, a hypervascularized area is observed in segment IV of the liver. (**b**) The RHA is preserved, and it arises from the SMA. RHA: Right Hepatic Artery; LHA: Left Hepatic Artery; CT: Celiac Trunk; SMA: Superior Mesenteric Artery; GDA: Gastroduodenal Artery; SA: Splenic Artery

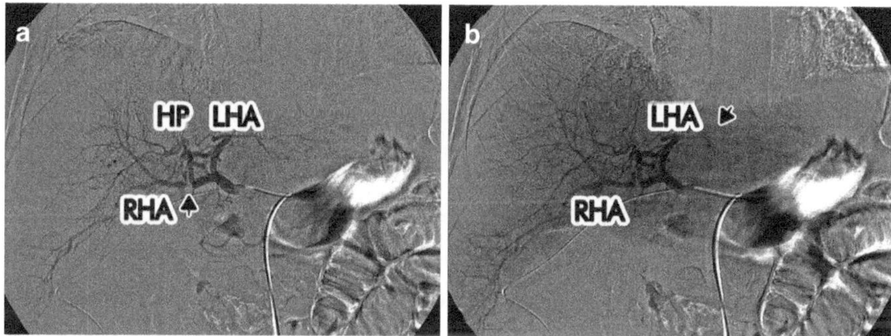

Fig. 10.7 Digital angiography case II. (**a**) The black arrow points a segmental obstruction of the RHA which presents intrahepatic anastomoses through the HP that distally vascularize the right hepatic lobe. The LHA is intact. (**b**) Black arrow shows an appropriate washout of the liver in a delayed phase. The right hepatic lobe remains perfused. RHA: Right Hepatic Artery; LHA: Left Hepatic Artery; HP: hilar plexus

Conclusion

A comprehensive assessment of AVI in the setting of a BDI is mandatory to delineate the most appropriate reparative strategy and to estimate its prognosis.

Most of the time non-invasive methods such as a CT angiography with three-dimensional reconstruction suffice for a thorough assessment of the hepatic vasculature in these complex scenarios.

However, when there is uncertainty in the diagnosis of an AVI, indirect signs of an AVI are present, or a bleeding complication occurred, the role of the conventional angiography becomes a central player.

The most common AVI in the setting of a BDI is the RHA and is usually asymptomatic.

However, the higher the lesion, the more likely it is to affect the compensatory system and ultimately affect the arterial supply to the liver with their respective consequences.

References

1. Pulitanò C, Parks RW, Ireland H, Wigmore SJ, Garden OJ. Impact of concomitant arterial injury on the outcome of laparoscopic bile duct injury. Am J Surg. 2011;201:238–44.
2. Strasberg SM, Helton WS. An analytical review of vasculobiliary injury in laparoscopic and open cholecystectomy. HPB. 2011;13:1–14.
3. Koffron A, Ferrario M, Parsons W, Nemcek A, Saker M, Abecassis M. Failed primary management of iatrogenic biliary injury: incidence and significance of concomitant hepatic arterial disruption. Surgery. 2001;130:722–8; discussion 728–31.
4. Gupta N, Solomon H, Fairchild R, Kaminski DL. Management and outcome of patients with combined bile duct and hepatic artery injuries. Arch Surg. 1998;133:176–81.
5. Buell JF, Cronin DC, Funaki B, Koffron A, Yoshida A, Lo A, Leef J, Millis JM. Devastating and fatal complications associated with combined vascular and bile duct injuries during cholecystectomy. Arch Surg. 2002;137:703–8; discussion 708–10.
6. Wachsberg RH, Cho KC, Raina S. Liver infarction following unrecognized right hepatic artery ligation at laparoscopic cholecystectomy. Abdom Imaging. 1994;19:53–4.
7. Mercado MA, Domínguez I. Classification and management of bile duct injuries. World J Gastrointest Surg. 2011;3:43–8.
8. Balsara KP, Dubash C, Shah CR. Pseudoaneurysm of the hepatic artery along with common bile duct injury following laparoscopic cholecystectomy. A report of two cases. Surg Endosc. 1998;12:276–7.
9. Madanur MA, Battula N, Sethi H, Deshpande R, Heaton N, Rela M. Pseudoaneurysm following laparoscopic cholecystectomy. Hepatobiliary Pancreat Dis Int. 2007;6:294–8.
10. Machado NO, Al-Zadjali A, Kakaria AK, Younus S, Rahim MA, Al-Sukaiti R. Hepatic or cystic artery pseudoaneurysms following a laparoscopic cholecystectomy: a literature review of aetiopathogenesis, presentation, diagnosis and management. Sultan Qaboos Univ Med J. 2017;17:e135–46.
11. Dandekar U, Dandekar K, Chavan S. Right hepatic artery: a cadaver investigation and its clinical significance. Anat Res Int. 2015;2015:412595.
12. Schmidt SC, Settmacher U, Langrehr JM, Neuhaus P. Management and outcome of patients with combined bile duct and hepatic arterial injuries after laparoscopic cholecystectomy. Surgery. 2004;135:613–8.
13. Kageyama Y, Kokudo T, Amikura K, Miyazaki Y, Takahashi A, Sakamoto H. The arc of Buhler: special considerations when performing pancreaticoduodenectomy. Surg Case Rep. 2016;2:21.
14. McNulty JG, Hickey N, Khosa F, O'Brien P, O'Callaghan JP. Surgical and radiological significance of variants of Bühler's anastomotic artery: a report of three cases. Surg Radiol Anat. 2001;23:277–80.
15. Northover JM, Terblanche J. A new look at the arterial supply of the bile duct in man and its surgical implications. Br J Surg. 1979;66:379–84.

16. Shapiro AL, Robillard GL. The arterial blood supply of the common and hepatic bile ducts with reference to the problems of common duct injury and repair: based on a series of twenty-three dissections. Surgery. 1948;23:1–11.
17. Gunji H, Cho A, Tohma T, et al. The blood supply of the hilar bile duct and its relationship to the communicating arcade located between the right and left hepatic arteries. Am J Surg. 2006;192:276–80.
18. Redman HC, Reuter SR. Arterial collaterals in the liver hilus. Radiology. 1970;94:575–9.
19. Bengmark S, Rosengren K. Angiographic study of the collateral circulation to the liver after ligation of the hepatic artery in man. Am J Surg. 1970;119:620–4.
20. Plengvanit U, Chearanai O, Sindiivananda K, Damrongsak D, Tuchinda S, Viranuvatti V. Collateral arterial blood supply of the liver after hepatic artery ligation, angiographic study of twenty patients. Ann Surg. 1972;175:105–10.
21. Yeh BM, Liu PS, Soto JA, Corvera CA, Hussain HK. MR imaging and CT of the biliary tract. Radiographics. 2009;29:1669–88.
22. Horton KM, Talamini MA, Fishman EK. Median arcuate ligament syndrome: evaluation with CT angiography. Radiographics. 2005;25:1177–82.
23. de'Angelis N, Catena F, Memeo R, et al. 2020 WSES guidelines for the detection and management of bile duct injury during cholecystectomy. World J Emerg Surg. 2021;16:30.

Chapter 11
Postoperative Treatment

Ignacio Fuente and Martín de Santibañes

Introduction

Between 15% and 40% of BDI are diagnosed during the primary procedure. This variability is multifactorial, although the type of approach (open or laparoscopic), the circumstances of the surgery (elective or emergency), and the use of an IOC could weigh the balance towards an early or a more delayed diagnosis of a BDI [1, 2].

Nevertheless, the vast majority of BDIs are diagnosed during the postoperative phase significantly wavering the clinical scenario compared to the ones diagnosed during the primary surgery, and certainly changing the course of action [3].

Acute complications within the postoperative phase of BID are situations that must be attended to urgently. They are usually a result of disruption of the biliary integrity and its consequent leakage into the peritoneal cavity. If this bile leak remains localized, it would form an abdominal collection or a biloma. However, when the leak is not contained, it can extend to the whole peritoneal cavity and cause biliary peritonitis. In either case, these events can rapidly cause severe deterioration of the patient, ranging from sepsis, bacteremia, multiorgan failure, and death [4, 5].

I. Fuente
Upper GI and Bariatric Surgery Unit, General Surgery Service, Hospital Italiano de Buenos Aires, Buenos Aires, Argentina
e-mail: ignacio.fuente@hospitalitaliano.org.ar

M. de Santibañes (✉)
HPB Surgery and Liver Transplant Unit, Hospital Italiano de Buenos Aires, Buenos Aires, Argentina
e-mail: martin.desantibanes@hospitalitaliano.org.ar

J. Pekolj et al. (eds.), *Fundamentals of Bile Duct Injuries*,
https://doi.org/10.1007/978-3-031-13383-1_11

In calamitous cases, the acute phase may be starred by the presence of hepatic parenchymal ischemia secondary to a catastrophic associated vascular injury (AVI) (see Chaps. 9 and 10).

The long-term evolution of BDI will depend on the degree of the BDI, their eventual AVI, and their response to initial treatments [6].

Significant BDI will determine a partial or complete bile duct obstruction, that if left untreated will cause recurrent cholangitis and ultimately secondary biliary cirrhosis (SBC) requiring a liver transplant (LT) as a life-saving measure in the long run [7].

Treatment Overview

The main goal in the postoperative management of BDI is to *control sepsis* in the first instance and to convert an uncontrolled biliary leak into a controlled external biliary fistula to achieve optimal local and systemic control.

Definitive treatment to re-establish biliary continuity will be deferred once this primary goal is achieved and should not be obsessively pursued in the acute phase.

The factors that will determine the initial presentation of a patient with a BDI in the postoperative stage *are related to the time elapsed since the primary surgery, the type of injury, the mechanism of injury, and the overall general condition of the patient* [8]. Next, we are going to discuss each of these.

Mechanism of Injury

Thermal This is the most frequent. Thermal injuries have the peculiarity of progressing after they have been produced because they generate an ischemic effect on the affected tissue. The extent of the thermal injury is difficult to determine intraoperatively, and its delimitation is completed at a late stage. Because of this, it is recommended to defer the final repair for a minimum of 6–8 weeks or to perform bile duct resection prior to reconstruction.

Thus, it is clear that the recognition of a thermal mechanism of injury is essential as it is one of the main factors involved in the failure of an early biliary repair [9].

Metallic Clips A BDI can be produced by incorrect placement of clips secondary to misinterpretation of the anatomy or more frequently while performing blind hemostasis maneuvers to control a bleeder. This incident will result as a matter of course in cholestasis and jaundice secondary to extrinsic biliary stenosis.

Cold Section It can be caused by a sharp section with scissors or more rarely by injury from the transcystic choledocholithotomy intervention [10].

Septic Complications

Patients with septic complications usually manifest symptoms within the first hours or days after the BDI occurred. The clinical picture is characterized by fever, abdominal pain, hyperbilirubinemia, and signs of sepsis that may lead to multiorgan compromise.

Intra-abdominal abscesses, bilomas, biliary peritonitis, or even bile leakage through external drains can be present as well.

These situations put the patient's life at risk, so the treating team must act quickly and aggressively, focusing on the control of the septic condition. Establishing life support measures such as intravenous antibiotics and antifungals, resuscitation with crystalloids, and drainage of the septic source such as biliary peritonitis, biloma, abscess, or even the biliary tree in case of severe cholangitis is imperative [11].

Repair of the bile duct is not an emergency and should be deferred until the patient's condition improves [8]. In the interim, it is important to achieve control of the bile leak, improve local and general septic conditions, and the patient's nutritional status. Moreover, time will help in the delimitation of the margins of injury when a thermal mechanism was involved.

Currently, widely available imaging equipment and advanced interventional radiology techniques have great therapeutic precision with minimal invasion, for which they are considered first-line. The percutaneous approach to abdominal collections (abscess, biloma) is the best option for these kinds of patients (Fig. 11.1).

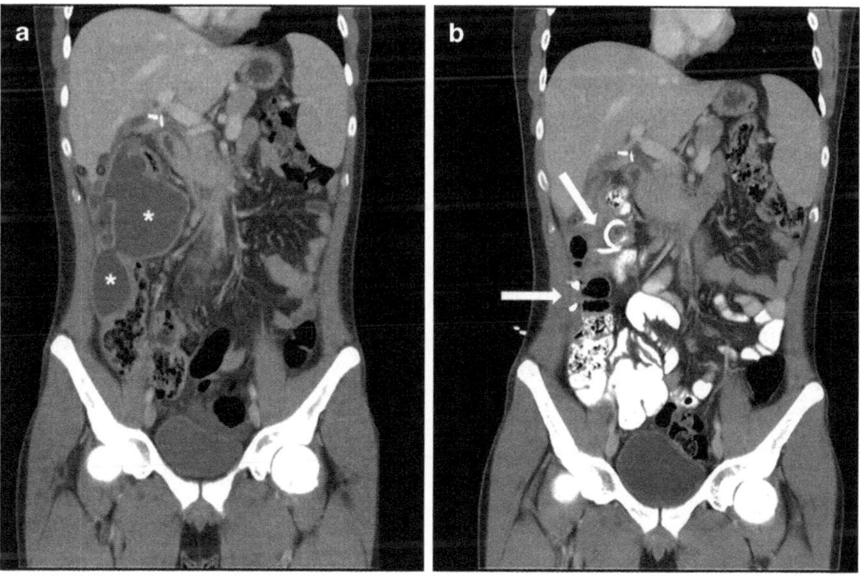

Fig. 11.1 (**a**) Coronal section of CT-scan demonstrating two abdominal fluid collections (marked with an asterisk) suspicious for biloma in a patient that underwent a laparoscopic cholecystectomy 7 days before. (**b**) Coronal section of CT-scan showing that the mentioned collection was drained (marked with black arrows)

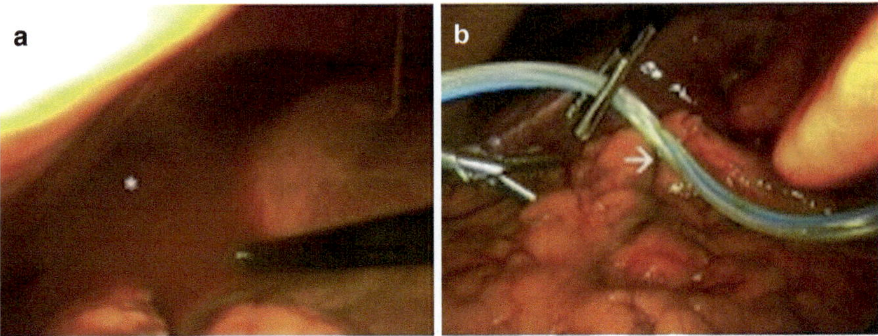

Fig. 11.2 Laparoscopic washout of a choleperitoneum (marked with asterisk). The arrow shows an abdominal drain that was being placed. (**a**) Intraoperative view of diffuse choleperitoneum. (**b**) A laparoscopic whas out was performed and abdominal drains were left in place

Surgical exploration of the abdominal cavity would be reserved for patients with possible peritonitis, without excluding the laparoscopic approach since it also permits a thorough exploration and washout of the abdomen [12, 13] (Fig. 11.2).

During the exploration, our recommendation in this scenario will always be conservative management of the BDI, leaving external drains at the level of the suspected injury and keeping adequately drained the regions of the abdomen that are difficult to access by percutaneous techniques (diaphragmatic domes and pelvic cul-de-sac).

Non-septic Complications

The most common complication is cholestasis and jaundice, which may or may not be associated with abdominal pain or cholangitis [14].

As a rule of thumb, high BD stenosis commonly requires percutaneous biliary drainage (PBD) (see Chap. 12) (Fig. 11.3).

Decompression of the biliary tree relieves jaundice and allows the type and extent of the injury to be defined [15].

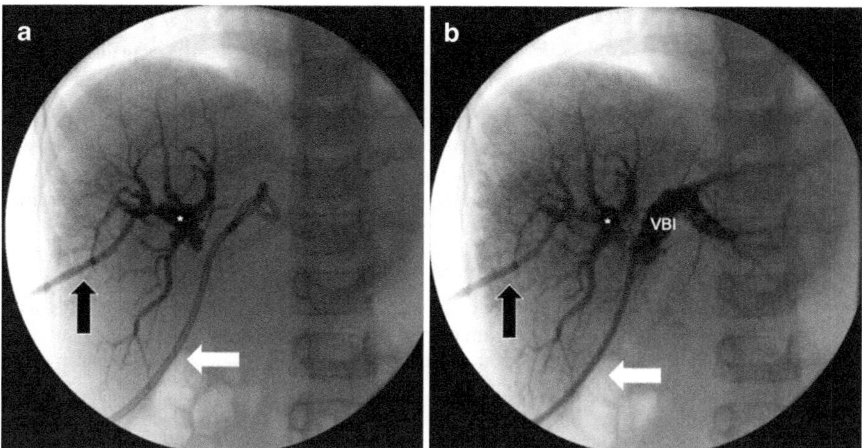

Fig. 11.3 Pediatric patient that presented with cholangitis 3 weeks after a cholecystectomy. Both left (LHD) and right hepatic duct (RHD) were compromised by a severe BDI. (**a**): Percutaneous transhepatic cholangiogram (PTC) at the right sided ducts (asterisk) and percutaneous biliary drainage (PBD) insertion (black arrow). No passage of contrast over the LHD is noted. The white arrow shows PBD in the LHD. (**b**) PTC at the RHD (asterisk) and PBD insertion (black arrow). The white arrow shows PBD in the LHD as well

ERCP would also have a role in the treatment of these patients. Leaks in the cystic duct and sometimes in the hepatic ducts can be treated by sphincterotomy and stent insertion that effectively decompresses the biliary tree (see Chap. 13).

Definitive Treatment

A BDI is considered a highly complex pathology, and its treatment must involve a multidisciplinary team integrated by surgeons, gastroenterologists, endoscopists interventional radiologists, social workers, physiotherapists, and dietitians to obtain the best results. Discussion about how and when to implement determining therapeutic approaches have to be done and tailored on a case-by-case basis to achieve the best long-term outcomes [16].

It is not unfrequent to see non-hepatobiliary surgeons managing these extremely complex cases, which ultimately can complicate even more the injury and compromise its definitive repair [17].

Pitt et al. demonstrated in 289 patients with BDI (Strasberg B-E), a more successful outcome for patients managed by hepatobiliary surgeons (88%) followed by endoscopists (76%) and interventional radiologists (50%). On the other hand, outcomes were worse in (a) patients treated endoscopically late (2–6 months) and (b) patients who underwent surgery 2–4 weeks after injury [18].

Interestingly, surgical and endoscopic management for the first 6–12 months following the injury remained significant predictors of success in multivariate analyses [19].

The results of endoscopic management of Strasberg B-E stenosis are not as good as those of reconstructive surgery.

The results of percutaneous treatment of bile duct stenosis are below those of surgery and endoscopy, with success rates of 50%. The percutaneous approach offers an option for patients who have previously been offered reconstructive surgery [20].

Treatment According to the Type of the Injury

- **Bile leaks from the *cystic duct* or from a *subvesical duct of Luschka*** (*Strasberg type A lesion*). These are accessory ducts that originate in the right hepatic lobe and have variable drainage into the bile duct (most frequently in the right hepatic or CBD).

  Postoperatively, depending on the patient's condition, treatment generally requires only drainage, either laparoscopically or percutaneously. They occasionally require an ERCP and sphincterotomy to decompress the biliary tree [21].
- *Injury to the right posterior hepatic duct (RPHD)*

  If the RPHD was clipped or ligated (*Strasberg type B lesion*), the patient will usually run an asymptomatic course producing atrophy of the affected segments. If the patient develops repeated cholangitis, with concomitant parenchymal atrophy there may be an indication for a hepatic lobectomy [22]. Otherwise, restoring the biliary tree continuity through a Roux-en-Y Hepaticojejunostomy (HJ) might be considered.

  If the posterior RPHD was divided *(Strasberg type C lesion)* there will be a biliary fistula, with the previously described manifestations. In these cases, primary suturing of the duct may be attempted, but in most cases an HJ over this compromised duct is definitive [23].

  If a stricture of the duct develops, percutaneous balloon angioplasty dilatation may be attempted and if unsuccessful, definitive treatment may require a liver resection [24].
- **Lateral common bile duct injury** *(Strasberg type D)*: This type of injury can be repaired by performing ERCP with stent insertion or percutaneous dilatation if the stenosis is short (such as in the case of an endobiliary instrumentation injury) or, if not effective, reconstruction through an HJ would be definitive [25].

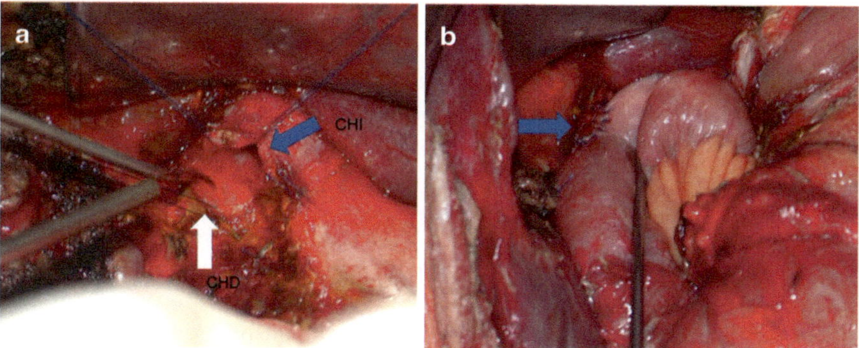

Fig. 11.4 Patient with complex BDI. (**a**): RHD is marked with the white arrow, and LHC with a blue arrow, being prepared for an anastomosis. (**b**) Hepaticojejunostomy (blue arrow)

- **In cases of complex lesions injuries such as *Strasberg type E***: The definitive treatment consists of performing an HJ. In cases of high stenosis (Bismuth type III and IV), exposure of the left hepatic duct (Hepp Couinaud operation), separate anastomosis of the hepatic ducts or of the sectoral collectors, or resection of hepatic segment IV B to expose the confluence of the hepatic ducts will be necessary [26] (Fig. 11.4).

To obtain good long-term results, it is necessary to perform the HJ with excellent technique. Technical failures are the main factor conditioning anastomotic strictures that manifest within a few months following the reconstruction and would require further therapies, like percutaneous balloon dilatations or eventually a re-do HJ [27].

In cases with a poor general condition, evidence of SBC and/or of portal hypertension, and very high stenosis, we recommend percutaneous treatment as first-line therapy (balloon dilatation without prosthesis placement). Otherwise, we prefer reoperation and anastomosis as described above.

Despite refined techniques, and related to the complexity of these injuries, the future of these patients is uncertain. Some will require several treatments and yet will eventually progress to CBS, where the only valid treatment would be a LT [28].

When Is the Best Time to Perform the Definitive Surgical Repair?

The best time to perform an HJ after a BID is a matter of continuous debate and depends on several factors. Academically, the timing is divided into three different opportunities within *1 week (early); 1–6 weeks (intermediate); 6 weeks–6 months (late).* However, there are several aspects to consider, other than time [29].

Immediate reconstruction is more likely feasible when the lesion is detected intraoperatively during cholecystectomy or in the very early postoperative period, since an early repair, whenever possible, allows for adequate anastomosis without associated complications and a related systemic inflammatory response [30].

When the injury is detected after the primary surgery, the timing of repair will depend on several factors such as sepsis, the patient's general condition, and the surgeon's training.

Adequate sepsis control is associated with fewer postoperative complications and a higher likelihood of successful repair; therefore it should be first and foremost guaranteed.

On the other hand, late repairs (after 6 weeks from the primary procedure) offer a less inflamed site, with more defined and adequately vascularized bile ducts and with control of the infection.

Repairs between 8 days and 6 weeks its been shown to increase the overall postoperative complications and failure rates of the reconstruction.

Therefore, decisions should be made multidisciplinary on a case-by-case basis, carefully weighing the risk and benefits of the different therapeutic options.

These concepts are summarized in Figs. 11.5 and 11.6.

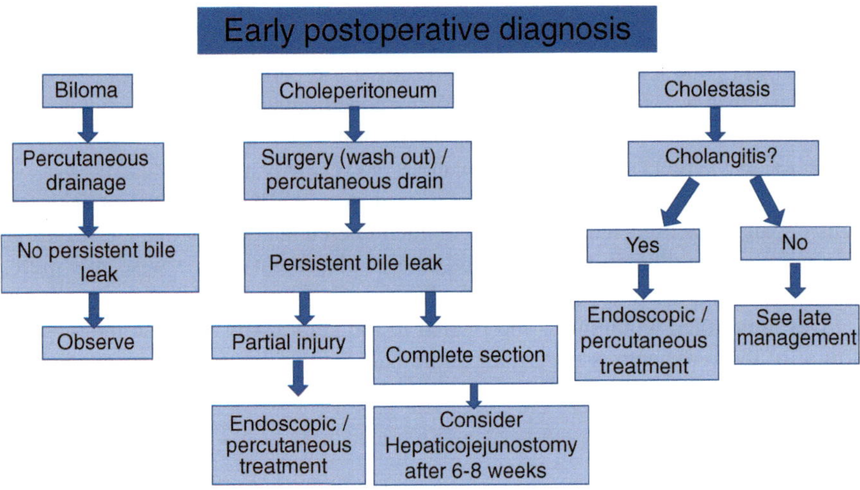

Fig. 11.5 Algorithm of early postoperative management

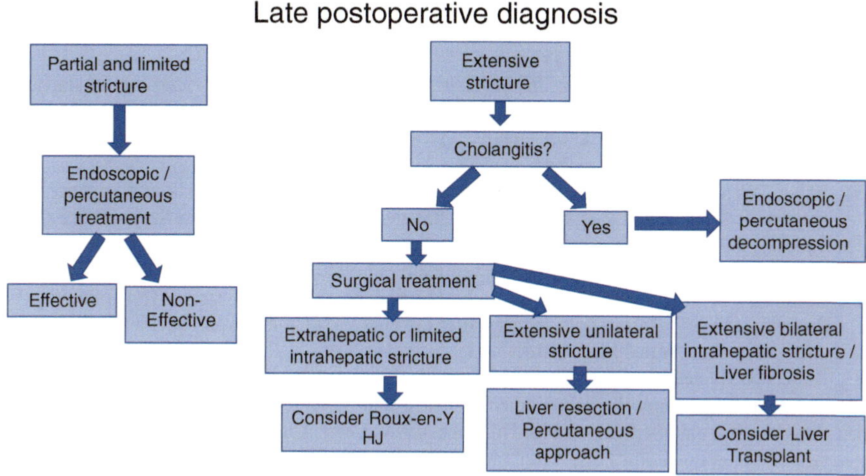

Fig. 11.6 Algorithm of late postoperative management

References

1. Buddingh KT, Nieuwenhuijs VB, van Buuren L, Hulscher JBF, de Jong JS, van Dam GM. Intraoperative assessment of biliary anatomy for prevention of bile duct injury: a review of current and future patient safety interventions. Surg Endosc. 2011;25:2449–61.
2. Wu J-S, Peng C, Mao X-H, Lv P. Bile duct injuries associated with laparoscopic and open cholecystectomy: sixteen-year experience. World J Gastroenterol. 2007;13:2374–8.
3. de'Angelis N, Catena F, Memeo R, et al. 2020 WSES guidelines for the detection and management of bile duct injury during cholecystectomy. World J Emerg Surg. 2021;16:30.
4. Lee CM, Stewart L, Way LW. Postcholecystectomy abdominal bile collections. Arch Surg. 2000;135:538–42; discussion 542–4.
5. Christoforidis E, Vasiliadis K, Goulimaris I, Tsalis K, Kanellos I, Papachilea T, Tsorlini E, Betsis D. A single center experience in minimally invasive treatment of postcholecystectomy bile leak, complicated with biloma formation. J Surg Res. 2007;141:171–5.
6. Buell JF, Cronin DC, Funaki B, Koffron A, Yoshida A, Lo A, Leef J, Millis JM. Devastating and fatal complications associated with combined vascular and bile duct injuries during cholecystectomy. Arch Surg. 2002;137:703–8; discussion 708–10.
7. Nordin A, Halme L, Mäkisalo H, Isoniemi H, Höckerstedt K. Management and outcome of major bile duct injuries after laparoscopic cholecystectomy: from therapeutic endoscopy to liver transplantation. Liver Transpl. 2002;8:1036–43.
8. Sulpice L, Garnier S, Rayar M, Meunier B, Boudjema K. Biliary cirrhosis and sepsis are two risk factors of failure after surgical repair of major bile duct injury post-laparoscopic cholecystectomy. Langenbeck's Arch Surg. 2014;399:601–8.
9. Portella AOV, Trindade MRM, Dias LZ, Goldenberg S, Trindade EN. Monopolar electrosurgery on the extrahepatic bile ducts during laparoscopic cholecystectomy: an experimental controlled trial. Surg Laparosc Endosc Percutan Tech. 2009;19:213–6.
10. Lau WY, Lai ECH, Lau SHY. Management of bile duct injury after laparoscopic cholecystectomy: a review. ANZ J Surg. 2010;80:75–81.

11. Sicklick JK, Camp MS, Lillemoe KD, et al. Surgical management of bile duct injuries sustained during laparoscopic cholecystectomy: perioperative results in 200 patients. Ann Surg. 2005;241:786–92; discussion 793–5.
12. Pekolj J, Drago J. Controversies in iatrogenic bile duct injuries. Role of video-assisted laparoscopy in the management of iatrogenic bile duct injuries. Cir Esp. 2020;98:61–3.
13. Gupta V, Jayaraman S. Role for laparoscopy in the management of bile duct injuries. Can J Surg. 2017;60:300–4.
14. Bauer TW, Morris JB, Lowenstein A, Wolferth C, Rosato FE, Rosato EF. The consequences of a major bile duct injury during laparoscopic cholecystectomy. J Gastrointest Surg. 1998;2:61–6.
15. Thompson CM, Saad NE, Quazi RR, Darcy MD, Picus DD, Menias CO. Management of iatrogenic bile duct injuries: role of the interventional radiologist. Radiographics. 2013;33:117–34.
16. Karanikas M, Bozali F, Vamvakerou V, Markou M, Memet Chasan ZT, Efraimidou E, Papavramidis TS. Biliary tract injuries after lap cholecystectomy-types, surgical intervention and timing. Ann Transl Med. 2016;4:163.
17. Butte JM, Hameed M, Ball CG. Hepato-pancreato-biliary emergencies for the acute care surgeon: etiology, diagnosis and treatment. World J Emerg Surg. 2015;10:13.
18. Pitt HA, Sherman S, Johnson MS, Hollenbeck AN, Lee J, Daum MR, Lillemoe KD, Lehman GA. Improved outcomes of bile duct injuries in the 21st century. Ann Surg. 2013;258:490–9.
19. Stewart L, Way LW. Laparoscopic bile duct injuries: timing of surgical repair does not influence success rate. A multivariate analysis of factors influencing surgical outcomes. HPB. 2009;11:516–22.
20. Fong ZV, Pitt HA, Strasberg SM, Loehrer AP, Sicklick JK, Talamini MA, Lillemoe KD, Chang DC, California Cholecystectomy Group. Diminished survival in patients with bile leak and ductal injury: management strategy and outcomes. J Am Coll Surg. 2018;226:568–576.e1.
21. Iida H, Matsui Y, Kaibori M, Matsui K, Ishizaki M, Hamada H, Kon M. Single-center experience with subvesical bile ducts (ducts of Luschka). Am Surg. 2017;83:e43–5.
22. Jabłońska B. Hepatectomy for bile duct injuries: when is it necessary? World J Gastroenterol. 2013;19:6348–52.
23. Singh H, Avudaiappan M, Yadav TD. Surgical management of sectoral bile duct injury after cholecystectomy - a case series. HPB. 2021;23:S365–6.
24. Li J, Frilling A, Nadalin S, Broelsch CE, Malago M. Timing and risk factors of hepatectomy in the management of complications following laparoscopic cholecystectomy. J Gastrointest Surg. 2012;16:815–20.
25. Kapoor VK. Post-cholecystectomy bile duct injury. Springer Nature; 2020.
26. Mercado MA, Chan C, Orozco H, Tielve M, Hinojosa CA. Acute bile duct injury. The need for a high repair. Surg Endosc. 2003;17:1351–5.
27. De Santibáñes E, Ardiles V, Pekolj J. Complex bile duct injuries: management. HPB. 2008;10:4–12.
28. Desantibanes E, Pekolj J, Mccormack L, Nefa J, Acuna J, Mattera J, Gadano A, Sivori J, Ciardullo M. 180 liver transplantation for intraoperative biliary tree injuries. Liver Transpl. 2000;6:C45.
29. Schreuder AM, Nunez Vas BC, Booij KAC, van Dieren S, Besselink MG, Busch OR, van Gulik TM. Optimal timing for surgical reconstruction of bile duct injury: meta-analysis. BJS Open. 2020;4:776–86.
30. Iannelli A, Paineau J, Hamy A, Schneck A-S, Schaaf C, Gugenheim J. Primary versus delayed repair for bile duct injuries sustained during cholecystectomy: results of a survey of the Association Francaise de Chirurgie. HPB. 2013;15:611–6.

Chapter 12
The Role of Percutaneous Procedures

Sung Ho Hyon and Pablo Huespe

Introduction

A Bile Duct Injury (BDI) is a highly complex pathology. The diversity of the mechanisms of injury involved, their location of varying severity in the biliary tree, and the different forms of presentation can make their integrated management very challenging.

Image-guided percutaneous procedures have a key role in both the description of the injuries and their treatment. In the latter case, they can be used either as a bridge procedure (prior to restorative surgery) or as definitive treatment.

Clinical Presentation and Clinical Indication

The clinical presentation varies according to the type and extent of the injury, the mechanism of injury, the time elapsed, and the general condition of the patient.

Symptoms resulting from unrecognized BDI during surgery may present days, weeks, or even years after the primary surgical procedure. Early symptoms derive from the presence of choleperitoneum, biloma, cholangitis, or hemorrhage in cases with associated vascular injury.

In our institution, in the case of a BDI not recognized during surgery, presenting cholangitis or biliary fistula in the following days, we perform percutaneous

S. H. Hyon (✉) · P. Huespe
Image-Guided Minimally Invasive Surgery Unit, Hospital Italiano de Buenos Aires, Buenos Aires, Argentina

J. Pekolj et al. (eds.), *Fundamentals of Bile Duct Injuries*,
https://doi.org/10.1007/978-3-031-13383-1_12

transhepatic cholangiogram/percutaneous biliary drainage (PTC/PBD) to improve local conditions and defer surgical treatment for 6–8 weeks [1]. Accordingly, a PBD may be routinely performed and left in place until definitive repair surgery, at which time it may be replaced with a transanastomotic silastic tube that functions as a guardian.

Abscesses and Bilomas

Percutaneous treatment is mandatory. This approach solves practically 100% of cases, even in patients with multiple collections. The presence of generalized choleperitoneum usually requires surgical treatment.

Cholangitis

Percutaneous bile duct drainage is usually effective in the vast majority of injuries, especially the following, according to the Strasberg classification [2].

Grade B Injuries

In this type of injury, there is ligation of an aberrant hepatic duct, usually, the right posterior duct (RPD). If the drained segment is small, many of these patients evolve asymptomatically and with atrophy of the corresponding segment. In those patients who progress with cholangitis, percutaneous drainage of the affected segment and subsequent reconstruction with a definitive hepaticojejunostomy is indicated.

Grade C Injuries

Grade C injuries include those injuries with transection of an aberrant duct without communication with the Common Bile Duct (CBD). This type of injury, which cannot be approached endoscopically, tends to occur especially in patients with aberrant RHD and/or low implantation of it.

Grade E Injuries

These types of injuries present as complete injuries to the CBD. In patients with injury to the CBD or with an indemnity of the biliary confluence (Grades E1 and E2), it is enough to insert an external drain, proximal to the site of the injury. In cases of E3, E4, and E5 injuries, it is necessary to place bilateral access drains.

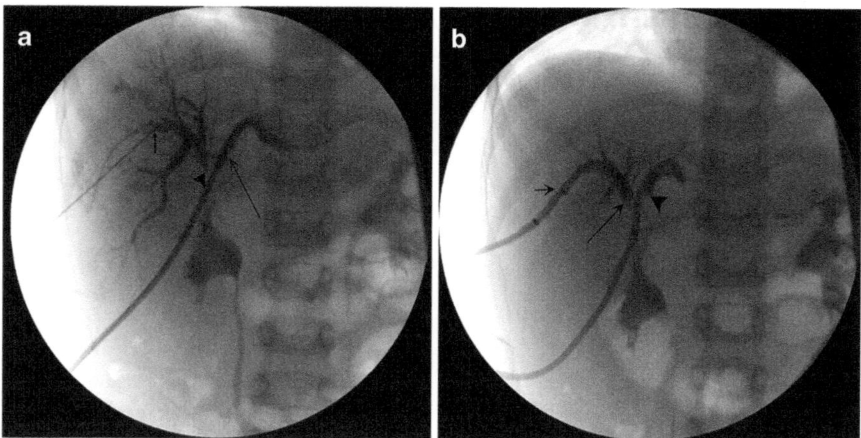

Fig. 12.1 A 5-year-old patient, with a complete section of the CBD, referred to our institution with surgical drainage offered to the left biliary tract. Cholangiogram showed stenosis of the hepatic confluence, and replacement of the left drainage and PBD of the right bile duct were performed. (**a**) Cholangiogram and puncture with a 22 Ga Chiba needle through the RPD (short arrow, Chiba needle in the right bile duct; arrowhead, stenosis; long arrow, drainage in the left bile duct). (**b**) With both drains (short arrow, drainage in right bile duct; long arrow, stenosis; arrowhead, drainage in the left bile duct)

The PBD is initially performed as a temporary treatment and may be converted to transanastomotic drainage during definitive surgical repair in patients with poor bile duct dilatation.

In patients with severe sepsis, it is advisable to drain the bile duct with as little manipulation as possible, minimizing contrast flushing and instrumentation. In these cases, it is advisable to place an external drain, which can later be replaced by an internal-external drain in those patients who require it (Fig. 12.1).

Stenosis After Hepaticojejunostomy (HJ)

The presence of an HJ makes the endoscopic approach extremely difficult, if not impossible, for anatomical reasons.

In this setting, percutaneous procedures are the treatment of choice. After placing a PBD, there are different treatment options. The most used modality is percutaneous high-pressure balloon dilatation (usually performed in different sessions), although there is no consensus on the different technical aspects, such as the number of sessions, the interval between them, the duration of treatment, or the diameter of the balloon.

In the series of patients from the Hospital Italiano de Buenos Aires, in both adult and pediatric patients, the implementation of a three-session protocol was associated with a statistically significant increase in the HJ patency, which reached 90% at 1 year, compared to one or two sessions [3, 4].

According to different publications, the 5-year patency rates of percutaneous balloon dilatation vary between 33% and 90%. Other options include sustained dilatation with multiple drains, the use of coated metal stents, and more recently, the use of biodegradable stents. For these approaches, there is not yet strong evidence, generated by prospective, randomized protocols, to support their indication on a routine basis [5].

Diagnostic Methods

The purpose of imaging studies is to rule out the presence of collections or other associated surgical complications (e.g., vascular injuries) and to assess the location and extent of the injury in the bile duct. Moreover, they can serve as a guide for surgical procedures, all of which will help to establish the most appropriate therapeutic strategy.

The methods employed include Ultrasonography (US), Computed Tomography (CT-scan), Magnetic Resonance Imaging/Magnetic Resonance Cholangiopancreatography (MRI/MRCP); Percutaneous Transhepatic Cholangiogram (PTC), sinusography, nuclear scintigraphy, and angiography.

US and CT-scan with intravenous contrast are very useful to determine the presence of collections.

MRI/MRCP imaging is the most accurate method to assess the extent and the location of injuries in the bile duct.

If the patient has abdominal drains inserted, either into bilomas or into the biliary duct, the instillation of dye material through them under fluoroscopic guidance will reveal fistulous tracts, other collections, or may even be useful to perform a cholangiogram through the cavity. PTC is also very useful for characterizing the injuries, but given its technical complexity, it is performed in the context of a PBD and in those patients who arrive at a definitive surgical procedure with doubts about the anatomy, and not as an isolated diagnostic tool.

Hepatobiliary scintigraphy (e.g., with HIDA, iminodiacetic acid) may be useful in patients with a suspected Strasberg Grade C injury that could not be detected by other diagnostic methods. In these cases, it would show the aberrant duct without communication with the bile duct. However, as a result of advances in other imaging methods, scintigraphy has recently fallen into disuse.

Angiography is the most convenient study for cases with suspected vascular associated injuries, although CT with angiographic protocol is a less invasive method with similar results.

Equipment and Materials

To perform a PBD, a fluoroscopy imaging intensifier and US are essential. The availability of a multi-track tomograph is important for the drainage of bilomas or collections, especially those located in the retroperitoneum or the center of the abdomen and pelvis, where US is less useful.

Materials

A variety of items should be available, such as needles, guide wires, angiographic catheters, coaxial introducers, and drains.

Needles

For the drainage of collections, 18 Ga spinal puncture needles, which allow the passage of a 0.035″ guide wire, are very useful. Chiba needles, 22 Ga by 15 cm in length, through which 0.018″ wires pass, are essential to access the biliary tree.

Guiding Wires

For initial access to the bile duct with a Chiba needle, 0.018″ wires are required. Hydrophilic 0.035″ wires (Roadrunner from Cook Medical; Glidewire from Terumo) are particularly useful for negotiating bile duct stenosis and narrowing. Furthermore, different angiographic catheters (e.g., Kumpe, Cook Medical) can be used in conjunction to direct the guide wires. The 0.035″ Amplatz type metal wires (Boston Scientific) have a stronger body than the previous ones and are very useful for bile duct procedures requiring extra support.

Introducers

They allow the exchange of a 0.018″ guide wire for a 0.035″ wire. The most commonly used are the Neff introducer, the D'Agostino introducer, and the Check-Flo introducer (Cook Medical). The latter two also allow contrast to be inserted through a lateral port without the necessity of removing the guide wire.

Drains

It is advisable to use catheters with pig-tail-type internal fixation devices. For drainage of abscesses, collections, and as external biliary drainage, multipurpose drains can be employed. Biliary catheters have proximal and distal fenestrae, which are positioned proximal and distal to the site of stenosis and are used for the placement of internal-external bile duct drains.

Percutaneous Procedures

Drainage of Bilomas and Collections

These types of drainage can be performed under US or fluoroscopy or a combination of both. US is most useful for superficial collections or those with a good acoustic window. Multi-track tomography is more effective for retroperitoneal collections or those with a poor acoustic window, either due to gas or bone interposition. Furthermore, the use of fluoroscopic guidance to complement a puncture under US guidance can also be very useful.

The small gauge (22 Ga) Chiba needle is suitable for difficult to access collections because the risks of complications due to unwanted puncture of surrounding structures (vessels and organs) are greatly reduced. However, according to Seldinger's technique, it has the "disadvantage" of having to use an exchanger to progress a larger gauge guide wire before placing the drainage.

When the collection to be punctured is superficial, a 16 or 18 Ga spinal type needle can be employed. Once access to the collection (confirmed by imaging methods) is achieved, a 0.035″ guide wire is passed, and a multipurpose catheter is placed over it.

Other methods for accessing collections are the trocar and tandem puncture techniques. In the first case, the drain is mounted on a mandrel-needle with which the collection is punctured, the drain is pushed in and the mandrel is withdrawn, without the requirement to use guide wires. In the tandem technique, the collection is accessed with a fine, guiding needle and, once the correct position is confirmed, the collection is punctured with another needle parallel to the first one. The procedure is completed according to Seldinger's technique or, alternatively, the drain may be placed using the tandem technique.

At the Hospital Italiano de Buenos Aires, the Seldinger's technique is the most commonly used due to its safety and high efficacy.

Percutaneous Drainage of the Bile Duct

In order to access the right bile duct, a low right intercostal access under fluoroscopy is employed. The puncture site is commonly placed at the level of the mid-axillary line, in the lower portion of the right hepatic lobe, through the upper border of the corresponding rib. A 21–22 Ga Chiba needle is progressed towards the xiphoid appendix and then withdrawn slowly, while contrast material is injected until bile duct opacification is confirmed by fluoroscopy.

The left bile duct is approached with a Chiba needle through the epigastrium under ultrasonographic guidance using 3.5–5.0 MHz transducers (convex). The entry into a bile duct is also confirmed by opacification of the bile duct with contrast material. The left access is associated with some advantages over the right: puncture under direct vision of the bile duct, less pain, absence of pleural injury, feasibility even in the presence of ascites, and, according to an analysis by our working group, less irradiation.

In both approaches, if the accessed duct is sufficiently peripheral to be able to place a drain, a 0.018″ guide wire is introduced, followed by a Neff or D'Agostino type introducer. Subsequently, the wire is exchanged for another 0.035″ wire, the tract is dilated and finally, the drain is placed, assuring the desired position by fluoroscopy.

Percutaneous Bile Duct Dilatation and Stent Placement, lithotripsy

High bile duct stenosis and stenosis of an HJ reconstruction are indications for percutaneous management. The most used treatment modality is percutaneous high-pressure balloon dilatation. As explained above, there is no consensus on the number of dilatations to be performed or the size of the balloon. In a recent analysis in our department, which included 46 patients with hepaticojejunal anastomotic stenosis, treated with three dilatation sessions vs. one or two sessions, we observed that, with three sessions, the patency of the anastomosis at 1 year was 90% vs. 50%, respectively, resulting in a statistically significant difference. We used 10 mm × 40 mm balloons, inflated to 6–8 atmospheres with a pressure syringe, for a duration of 5 min with a three-minute interval, repeated 3 times in each session. We recommend inserting the balloon inside an introducer, as the irregular surface of the balloon can injure the liver entrance, causing a bile leak.

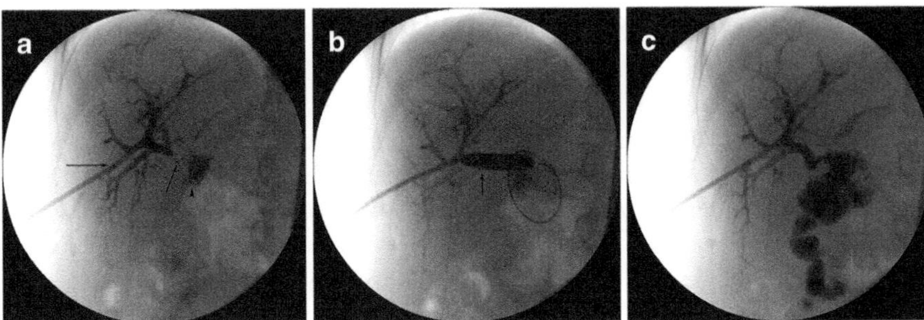

Fig. 12.2 32-year-old woman, with an HJ due to BDI which evolved with stenosis. PBD and subsequent dilatation with a 10 × 40 mm balloon were indicated. (**a**) Cholangiogram through a Cook Medical Check-Flo introducer (long arrow, introducer; short arrow, stenosis; arrowhead, the loop of the jejunum). (**b**) Balloon dilatation (arrow). (**c**) Result after dilatation

After the first session we keep an internal/external drain, an external drain in the second session, and after the last session, a smallbore, silastic catheter, which we remove after 10 days if the patient shows good clinical evolution (Fig. 12.2).

Rendez-vous

This is a combined percutaneous-endoscopic approach, which may be useful in cases with complete bile duct injury. These patients often have clips at the injured ends and a cavity between them, which prevents the use of internal/external drainage or endoscopic treatment. Moreover, a biliary fistula often coexists in the case of cholangitis.

Using the *Rendez-Vous* technique, a guide wire is passed from the percutaneous access through the proximal end of the bile duct to be collected in the perilesional cavity by an endoscopically advanced snare. In this way, once the bile duct has been reconnected, an internal/external drain can be placed from the percutaneous access, allowing the bile duct to be drained and the biliary fistula to be treated at the same time. Then, once a tract has been established, treatment can be continued endoscopically, either temporarily or permanently, by placing plastic stents (Fig. 12.3).

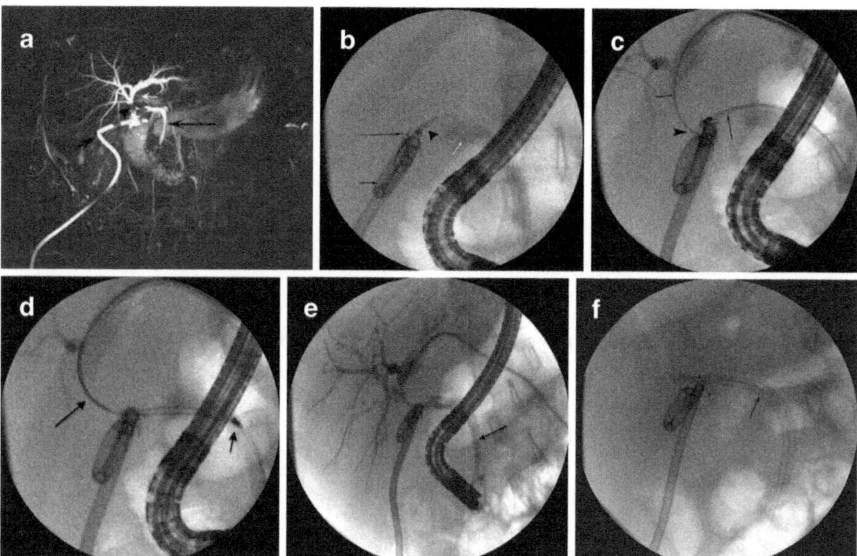

Fig. 12.3 A 30-year-old patient with a complete section of the CBD. Clips are observed at the level of the distal segment. The patient developed cholangitis and bile leak (through the surgical drainage). (**a**) MRCP, showing stenosis at the level of the hepatic duct confluence (arrowhead), the proximal CBD (white arrow), the distal CBD (long black arrow), and the drain at the surgical site (short black arrow). (**b**) ERCP showing a metallic clip in the area, and progression of the guide wire into the abdominal cavity (short black arrow, abdominal drainage; arrowhead, clip; long black arrow, hydrophilic guide wire; white arrow, distal bile duct). (**c**) PTC. With the assistance of a Kumbe angiographic catheter (short arrow), an attempt is made to pass the guide wire (arrowhead) into the distal CBD, without success. The guide wire is visible in the abdominal cavity, where the multipurpose drain is located. A snare was introduced endoscopically to perform the Rendez-vous (long arrow). (**d**) Percutaneous-endoscopic Rendez-vous procedure, in which the percutaneous guide wire (long arrow) is trapped with a snare advanced endoscopically (short arrow) and pulled into the distal CBD. (**e**) Once the guide wire has been passed into the duodenum, an internal/external drain is placed (arrow). (**f**) At a later stage, the internal/external drain was removed, and two plastic stents were placed endoscopically (arrow)

Complications

The complication rate after percutaneous bile duct drainage is 2.5% [6].

The most frequent complications include pain, bacteremia, and hyperamylasemia. More serious complications include haemobilia, cholangitis, pancreatitis, hemoperitoneum, bile leak, and pleural complications.

Many of these complications can be avoided by adequate preoperative planning and standardization of procedures. In patients with sepsis prior to drainage, minimal manipulation and placement of an external (rather than internal-external) drain are recommended, minimizing the risk of cholangitis and pancreatitis.

In right accesses, high, cephalad access points should be avoided, and the diaphragmatic dome should be observed under fluoroscopy throughout the procedure. The correct positioning of internal/external drainage fenestrae and the use of plastic introducers for balloon dilatation instrumentation may decrease the incidence of a bile leak.

Conclusions

BDI is a complex problem that requires a multidisciplinary approach for appropriate treatment. Initial damage control, including drainage of collections and bile duct decompression, allows control of the septic sites that determine the severity of the patient. Thus, image-guided percutaneous surgery offers a variety of essential tools for the initial recovery of the critical patient, enabling definitive surgical treatment to be performed electively. Furthermore, the percutaneous approach may result in the definitive treatment of many of these injuries and the complications arising from their surgical repair.

References

1. de Santibáñes E, Ardiles V, Pekolj J. Complex bile duct injuries: management. HPB (Oxford). 2008;10(1):4–12.
2. Strasberg SM, Hertl M, Soper NJ. An analysis of the problem of biliary injury during laparoscopic cholecystectomy. J Am College Surg. 1995;180(1):101–25.
3. Czerwonko ME, Huespe P, Mazza O, de Santibanes M, Sanchez-Claria R, Pekolj J, Ciardullo M, de Santibanes E, Hyon SH. Percutaneous biliary balloon dilation: impact of an institutional three-session protocol on patients with benign anastomotic strictures of hepatojejunostomy. Dig Surg. 2018;35(5):397–405.
4. Oggero AS, Bruballa RC, Huespe PE, de Santibañes M, Sanchez Claria R, Boldrini G, D'Agostino D, Pekolj J, de Santibañes E, Hyon SH. Percutaneous balloon dilatation for hepaticojejunostomy stricture following pediatric liver transplantation. Long-term results of an institutional "three-session protocol". Cardiovasc Intervent Radiol. 2021. https://doi.org/10.1007/s00270-021-03000-2.
5. Cantwell CP, Pena CS, Gervais DA, Hahn PF, Dawson SL, Mueller PR. Thirty years experience with balloon dilation of benign postoperative biliary strictures: long-term outcomes. Radiology. 2008;249(3):1050–7.
6. Saad WEA, Wallace MJ, Wojak JC, Kundu S, Cardella JF. Quality improvement guidelines for percutaneous transhepatic cholangiography, biliary drainage, and percutaneous cholecystostomy. J Vasc Interv Radiol. 2010;21(6):789–95.

Chapter 13
Role of Endoscopic Procedures

Carlos Macías Gómez and Federico Marcaccio

Introduction

From the endoscopist point of view, BDI usually present to us as bile leaks (0.5–3% of cholecystectomies), or as a stricture (0.2–0.5%) [1].

Once these events occur, they have a major impact on the morbidity, mortality, and quality of life of the affected patients [2].

Endoscopic Management of Bile Leak

Until a few years ago, surgical treatment was the primary approach to manage bile leaks that occurred after the intervention on the biliary tree. However, the treatment of these bile leaks has evolved using mini-invasive procedures such as endoscopic retrograde cholangiopancreatography (ERCP) associated with sphincterotomy and endobiliary stenting, at the point that it became one of the first-line therapies [3].

One of the goals of the endoscopic treatment is to decrease or eliminate the pressure gradient between the duodenal lumen and the biliary tree, directing the bile flow in a transpapillary direction into the duodenum and preventing or minimizing the outflow of bile through the site of the leak, which eventually leads to overheal the leaking site. This is achieved by conducting a biliary sphincterotomy (papillotomy) followed by the insertion of a prosthesis (stents), in which the proximal end should be located above the site of the leak [4].

C. Macías Gómez (✉)
Gastroenterlogy Department, Hospital Italiano de Buenos Aires, Buenos Aires, Argentina
e-mail: carlos.macias@hospitalitaliano.org.ar

F. Marcaccio
Páncreas Unit, Sanatorio Las Lomas, Buenos Aires, Argentina

J. Pekolj et al. (eds.), *Fundamentals of Bile Duct Injuries*,
https://doi.org/10.1007/978-3-031-13383-1_13

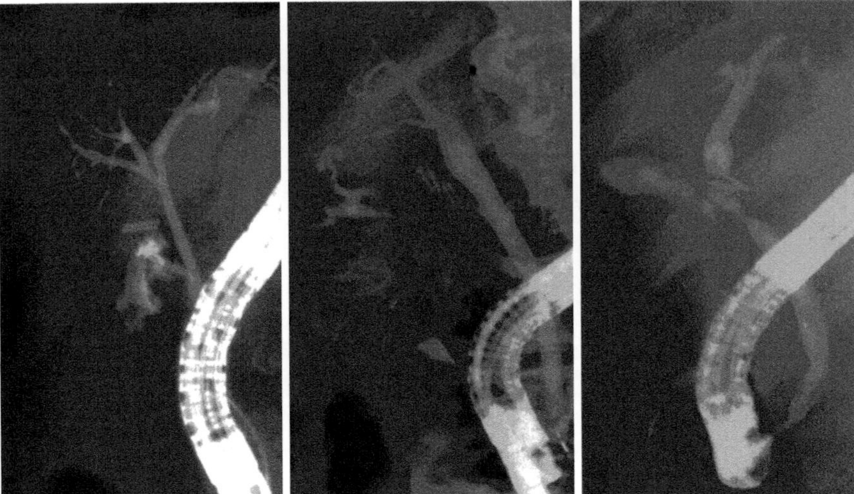

Fig. 13.1 ERCP Cholangiogram demonstrating bile leaks from the cystic duct stump; from a subvesical duct of Luschka draining in a right posterior duct, and from the right hepatic stump after right hepatectomy from left to right, respectively

The most common site of bile leaks varies according to the different published series, although they are generally reported at the level of the cystic duct stump. This is followed in decreasing order by the subvesical ducts (of Luschka) and the common bile duct (CBD) [5, 6] (Fig. 13.1).

Classifying bile leaks according to their severity is useful for the final decision on the endoscopic approach and has implications for the outcomes after endoscopic therapy. Bile leaks are classified as a "*high-grade*" when they become evident on fluoroscopy before a complete contrast filling of the biliary tree, while "*low-grade*" require complete filling of the entire biliary tree before becoming evident on fluoroscopic imaging [7].

The classic initial endoscopic approach consists of performing a sphincterotomy and inserting a 10 French diameter plastic prosthesis with its proximal end located over the site of the leak. Therapeutic success with this approach will be achieved in the majority of patients (≥90%) [8].

In the case of a persistent bile leak, a secondary cause must be evaluated (multiple leaking sites, associated stenosis, stones, etc.). Only if these causes have been ruled out, the leak will be considered "refractory" [9].

The endoscopic approach to these refractory bile leaks must be approached on a case-by-case basis, with two types of rescue strategy:

(a) *Insertion of multiple endobiliary stents.*
(b) *Temporary insertion of a fully covered metallic stent* [10].

Both approaches are usually highly effective for the resolution of bile leak, although no prospective randomized studies compare the two strategies.

Endoscopic Management of Biliary Strictures

Approximately 10% of postoperative biliary stenosis manifest within the first week after the primary surgery, while 70–80% are diagnosed after 6–12 months after surgery. The clinical presentation is variable and can manifest as cholestasis with or without symptoms, as recurrent cholangitis with stone formation, and in extreme cases, as Secondary Biliary Cirrhosis (SBC) if left untreated for a long time [11, 12].

Bismuth-Corlette Type I and II [13] *[See Chap. 6: Classification of Bile Duct Injuries]* strictures are the most frequently reported in clinical practice, and the most likely to be resolved by ERCP.

Diagnosis in the patients with clinical suspicion is made in the first instance with abdominal Ultrasound (US) which can suggest the level of obstruction in patients with a dilated bile duct. Magnetic resonance cholangiopancreatography (MRCP) is a non-invasive diagnostic method, which can accurately delineate the exact location of the stenosis, allowing us to schedule a definitive therapy [14]. It is currently the mandatory workup before proceeding to endoscopic treatment, to know with precision the level of the injury, and also the level of feasibility of successful endoscopic treatment.

Technique

Endoscopic treatment consists of successfully achieving two technical milestones:

1. *Passing through the stricture.*
2. *Dilating the full length of the stricture.*

Transposing a benign bile duct stricture is often a more challenging than transposing malignant stricture due to the asymmetry of the stenosis, associated with the additional fibrotic component, which ultimately makes it thinner and narrower. This requires the use of thin hydrophilic guiding wires (0.021 or 0.018 inches) with straight or curved tips, depending on the case, supported by straight catheters or with the possibility of modifying the exit axis of the guiding wire, as in sphincterotomes.

Manipulation of the guiding wire requires patience and being mindful that if excessive force is applied, could cause a formation of a false track.

In complex cases, the rectification of the duct below the stenosis may be necessary to change the axis of entry into the stricture, which can be achieved by insufflating and pulling with a balloon below the stricture, with changes in the patient's position, or the combination of both. Once the stenosis has been penetrated, the guiding wire can be replaced with a stiffer one to facilitate dilatation [15].

Biliary sphincterotomy is necessary when multiple plastic stents of larger caliber need to be placed in apposition, to avoid compression and difficult drainage of the pancreatic duct.

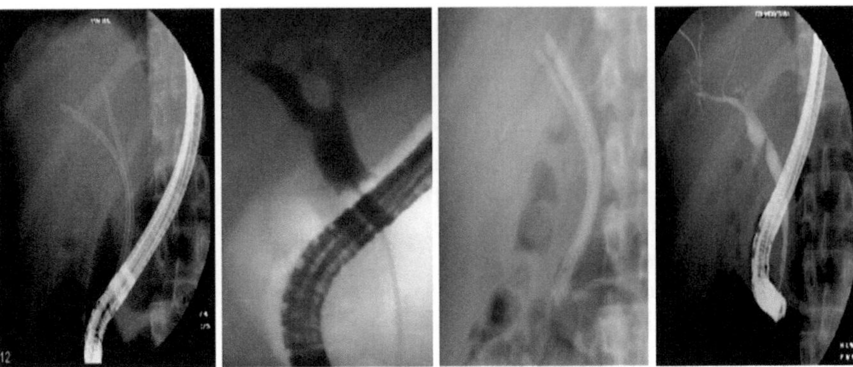

Fig. 13.2 Multiple plastic stent insertion through ERCP in the treatment of strictures related to BDI

The dilatation of the stricture has two purposes: in the first place to reopen the stenotic segment of the bile duct and maintain its distal drainage, and at the same time to maintain the stricture open in time [16].

Dilatation is performed using sequential hydrostatic balloons of 4-, 6-, and 8-mm diameter. The limit of dilatation should not exceed 1–2 mm of the duct diameter below the stricture. A dilatation itself is considered inadequate to preserve the caliber of the duct for a long time and is associated with a high rate of restenosis (>47%) [17]. In contrast, stent placement keeps the stenosis open for long periods of time while allowing fibrosis "remodeling" and consolidation of the stenotic segment. In general, 10 or 11.5 French polyethylene plastic stents are inserted and replaced every 3–4 months with an increase in their number if necessary for a period of 1 year or more, with the ultimate purpose of the disappearance of the stricture, assessed by performing a balloon-blocked cholangiogram, which minimizes the possibility of restenosis and maintains the patency of the duct in the long term (90% after an average follow-up of 13.7 years) [18] (Fig. 13.2). However, the optimal number of stents and duration of treatment to maintain stenosis resolution has not yet been established.

Recently, self-expandable metallic stents have been used as an alternative in BDIs. Their larger luminal diameter (8 and 10 mm) makes them an attractive alternative to single or multiple plastic stents [19].

Metallic stents can be uncovered, partially covered, and fully covered, although the first two are not recommended for treating these benign strictures due to ductal hyperplasia and endoluminal tissue growth through the mesh, which complicates or prevents subsequent removal [20].

Fully covered bare-metal stents were designed to avoid this problem but have a greater tendency to migrate both proximally and/or distally, and this is associated with a higher rate of complications during the period they remain in situ [10].

In a recent multinational study evaluating the use of these stents in benign post-surgical strictures, the resolution rate was observed in 72.2% of patients ($n = 18$) treated, leaving the stents in situ for 10–12 months with a migration rate of 18%.

Adverse events in Endoscopic Treatment

Complications of endoscopic treatment are those related to the sphincterotomy per se and to adverse events that may occur during the period the stents remain in situ.

Complications of sphincterotomy occur quite early and include pancreatitis, hemorrhage, and perforation in a frequency similar to other therapeutic interventions in the bile duct for other indications such as the removal of choledochal lithiasis [21].

Meanwhile, adverse events observed from the presence of stents while therapy are those related to stent dysfunction which includes obstruction, migration, or occlusion in the case of plastic stents, and migration or obstruction by hyperplastic tissue growth at the ends or through the mesh of metallic stents [22].

The clinical manifestation of these dysfunctions is mainly acute cholangitis, which requires re-endoscopy for stent replacement or repositioning to ensure proper biliary drainage [23].

Our Experience at the Hospital Italiano de Buenos Aires

Between January 1999 and December 2016, 61 patients with BDIs were referred to our department for urgent or selective endoscopic treatment. These patients were included in a prospective database, and their medical records were reviewed to document clinical data and the surgical and endoscopic bile duct intervention they had received.

A total of 234 endoscopic procedures were performed in these 61 patients, the majority of BDIs resulted from laparoscopic cholecystectomy in 36 (59%) patients, secondary to liver resection in 22 (36%) patients, and open surgery in 3 (5%) patients. Patient demographics, type of surgery, and endoscopic treatment are summarized in Table 13.1.

The initial endoscopic approach consisted of a cholangiogram and documentation of the site of the bile leak and/or stricture (previously documented in most patients through MRCP) followed by insertion of a hydrophilic guiding wire overlapping the site of the lesion, and then placement of a 10 French diameter, 9 cm long plastic prosthesis with the proximal end located above (proximal) to the site of the leak. All patients had a prior biliary sphincterotomy.

Table 13.1 Demographics, results of endoscopic treatment and complications in patients treated with ERCP for BDIs at our institution

	Bile leak *n* = 39 (64%)	Stricture *n* = 22 (36%)	Total *n* = 61
Age; *median (range)*	56 (18–78)	56.5 (17–82)	56 (17–82)
Male; *n (%)*	20 (51)	8 (36)	28 (46)
Primary Surgery[a] *n (%)*			
Cholecystectomy	15 (39.4)	20 (91)	35 (58.4)
Liver resection	22 (58)	1 (4.5)	23 (38.3)
Other	1 (2.6)	1 (4.5)	2 (3.3)
Endoscopic treatment			
Sphincterotomy *n (%)*	4 (9)	2 (9)	
Sphincterotomy + stenting *n (%)*	35 (91)	20 (91)	
Number of stents; median *(range)*	1 (0–1)	1 (0–5)	
Lapse until resolution (months) *median (range)*	2 (0.75–12)	5 (2–12)	
Results			
Treatment failure *n(%)*	1 (2.6)	2 (9)	
Complications *n(%)*	5 (13)	3 (14)	8 (13)
• Cholangitis	2	2	4
• Hyperamylasemia	1	0	1
• Pancreatitis	0	1	1
• Persistent leak	1	0	1
• Death[b]	1	0	1

IQR interquartile range
[a]*not available in 1 patient*
[b]*Death 48 h post procedure due to ongoing sepsis*

Patients with biliary stenosis (secondary to metallic clips, thermal injury) required sequential pre-dilation of the stenosis with biliary dilatation balloons of 4 and 6 mm diameter in the first procedure, and 8 and 10 mm diameter in successive procedures, increasing the number of stents at each replacement. At each stent replacement procedure (every 3–4 months), the caliber of the duct at the site of the stricture was re-evaluated by balloon-blocked cholangiogram, and the treatment was considered completed when the morphological disappearance of the stenosis was verified. The results of the endoscopic treatment in terms of duration, the maximum number of stents used, and complications during the treatment period are summarized in Table 13.1.

In the long-term follow-up, only two patients with a stricture had a recurrence within 3 years upon completion of endoscopic treatment. These patients who declined further endoscopic therapies opted for surgical treatment. The results of this follow-up are shown in Fig. 13.3.

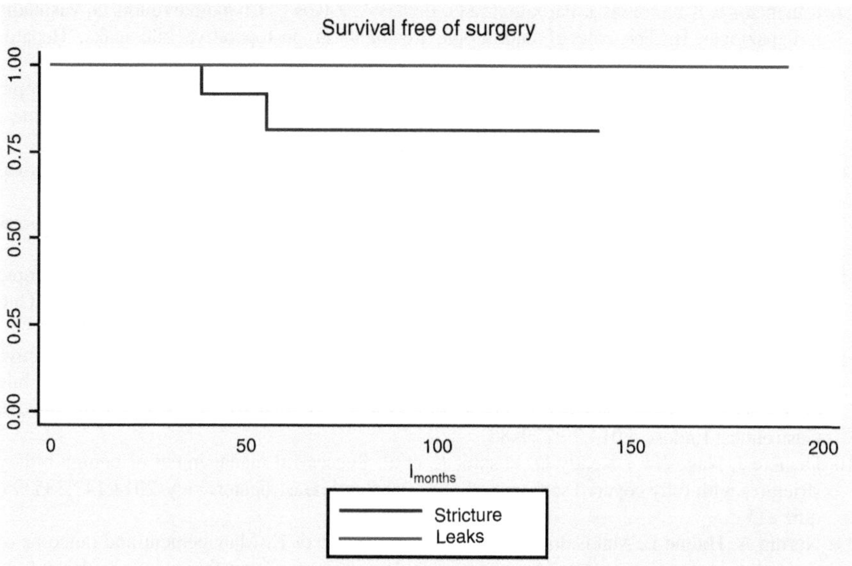

Fig. 13.3 Long-term follow-up of patients with BDIs that underwent ERCP + multiple plastic stenting

Conclusions

The endoscopic approach of the complications of a BDI such as bile leaks and/or strictures is essential. An aggressive approach using multiple plastic stents currently has the strongest evidence of long-term resolution of these benign strictures [24].

Metallic stents have gained great acceptance in recent years; however, studies with larger populations are needed to establish their real effectiveness in this type of stenosis.

In complex cases, in the therapeutic management of this pathology, the complementation of endoscopy with percutaneous procedures *(Rendez-Vous)* is a valid alternative [25] [*See Chap. 12 "role of percutaneous procedures"].*

References

1. Luigiano C, Iabichino G, Mangiavillano B, et al. Endoscopic management of bile duct injury after hepatobiliary tract surgery: a comprehensive review. Minerva Chir. 2016;71:398–406.
2. Booij KAC, de Reuver PR, van Dieren S, van Delden OM, Rauws EA, Busch OR, van Gulik TM, Gouma DJ. Long-term impact of bile duct injury on morbidity, mortality, quality of life, and work related limitations. Ann Surg. 2018;268:143–50.
3. de'Angelis N, Catena F, Memeo R, et al. 2020 WSES guidelines for the detection and management of bile duct injury during cholecystectomy. World J Emerg Surg. 2021;16:30.

4. Katsinelos P, Kountouras J, Paroutoglou G, Beltsis A, Zavos C, Chatzimavroudis G, Vasiliadis I, Papaziogas B. The role of endoscopic treatment in postoperative bile leaks. Hepato-Gastroenterology. 2006;53:166–70.
5. Kaffes AJ, Hourigan L, De Luca N, Byth K, Williams SJ, Bourke MJ. Impact of endoscopic intervention in 100 patients with suspected postcholecystectomy bile leak. Gastrointest Endosc. 2005;61:269–75.
6. Cortes N, Sabogal JC. Surgical importance of Duct of Luschka on bile duct leak: empirical review of literature. HPB. 2018;20:S167.
7. Agarwal N, Sharma BC, Garg S, Kumar R, Sarin SK. Endoscopic management of postoperative bile leaks. Hepatobiliary Pancreat Dis Int. 2006;5:273–7.
8. de Reuver PR, Rauws EA, Vermeulen M, Dijkgraaf MGW, Gouma DJ, Bruno MJ. Endoscopic treatment of post-surgical bile duct injuries: long term outcome and predictors of success. Gut. 2007;56:1599–605.
9. Canena J, Liberato M, Coutinho AP, Marques I, Romão C, Veiga PM, Neves BC. Predictive value of cholangioscopy after endoscopic management of early postcholecystectomy bile duct strictures with an increasing number of plastic stents: a prospective study (with videos). Gastrointest Endosc. 2014;79:279–88.
10. Devière J, Nageshwar Reddy D, Püspök A, et al. Successful management of benign biliary strictures with fully covered self-expanding metal stents. Gastroenterology. 2014;147:385–95. quiz e15
11. Nordin A, Halme L, Mäkisalo H, Isoniemi H, Höckerstedt K. Management and outcome of major bile duct injuries after laparoscopic cholecystectomy: from therapeutic endoscopy to liver transplantation. Liver Transpl. 2002;8:1036–43.
12. De Santibáñes E, Ardiles V, Pekolj J. Complex bile duct injuries: management. HPB. 2008;10:4–12.
13. Bismuth H. Postoperative strictures of the bile duct. Biliary Tract Clin Surg Int. 1982;5:209–18.
14. Reddy S, Lopes Vendrami C, Mittal P, Borhani AA, Moreno CC, Miller FH. MRI evaluation of bile duct injuries and other post-cholecystectomy complications. Abdom Radiol (NY). 2021;46:3086–104.
15. Pitt HA, Kaufman SL, Coleman J, White RI, Cameron JL. Benign postoperative biliary strictures. Operate or dilate? Ann Surg. 1989;210:417–25. discussion 426–7
16. Costamagna G, Pandolfi M, Mutignani M, Spada C, Perri V. Long-term results of endoscopic management of postoperative bile duct strictures with increasing numbers of stents. Gastrointest Endosc. 2001;54:162–8.
17. Baillie J. Endoscopic approach to the patient with bile duct injury. Gastrointest Endosc Clin N Am. 2013;23:461–72.
18. Draganov P, Hoffman B, Marsh W, Cotton P, Cunningham J. Long-term outcome in patients with benign biliary strictures treated endoscopically with multiple stents. Gastrointest Endosc. 2002;55:680–6.
19. Gabelmann A, Hamid H, Brambs HJ, Rieber A. Metallic stents in benign biliary strictures: long-term effectiveness and interventional management of stent occlusion. AJR Am J Roentgenol. 2001;177:813–7.
20. Park J-S, Lee SS, Song TJ, Park DH, Seo D-W, Lee SK, Han S, Kim M-H. Long-term outcomes of covered self-expandable metal stents for treating benign biliary strictures. Endoscopy. 2016;48:440–7.
21. Pawa S, Al-Kawas FH. ERCP in the management of biliary complications after cholecystectomy. Curr Gastroenterol Rep. 2009;11:160–6.
22. Uzer M, Hawes RH. Endoscopic retrograde cholangiography and laparoscopic cholecystectomy: stones, stents and sphincterotomy. Baillieres Clin Gastroenterol. 1993;7:921–40.

23. Bonnel DH, Liguory CL, Lefebvre JF, Cornud FE. Placement of metallic stents for treatment of postoperative biliary strictures: long-term outcome in 25 patients. AJR Am J Roentgenol. 1997;169:1517–22.
24. Vitale GC, Tran TC, Davis BR, Vitale M, Vitale D, Larson G. Endoscopic management of postcholecystectomy bile duct strictures. J Am Coll Surg. 2008;206:918–23. discussion 924–5
25. Vidovszky AA, Qafiti F, El Haddi SJ, Doukides T, Hus N, Genuit T. The use of percutaneous-endoscopic rendezvous stenting in a patient with bile duct injury after cholecystectomy—and a unique complication requiring secondary endoscopic intervention. J Surg Case Rep. 2021;2021:rjab119.

Chapter 14
Role of Minimally Invasive Surgery (MIS)

Jeremias Goransky and Guillermo Arbues

Minimally invasive surgery (MIS) indications, along different stages of bile duct injury (BDI), have significantly increased in recent years. Its application can be divided into two broad groups: intraoperative diagnosis and contemporization of BDIs, and treatment of the choleperitoneum (which can be conducted by the general/primary surgeon).

Intraoperative Diagnosis and Contemporization

Whenever a BDI is suspected, an IOC should be performed in order to define the biliary anatomy and avoid further dissection resulting in devascularization of any segment of the biliary tree [1] (Fig. 14.1).

The correct interpretation of IOC is easier when the surgeon performs it regularly and has acquired experience in recognizing all sectors of the biliary tree, as well as recognizing the broad spectrum of injuries that can occur and their respective cholangiographic presentation [2, 3].

If this confirms the diagnosis of BDI and the surgeon has no experience in complex biliary reconstructions, the injury should be *"contemporized."*

In this case scenario, there is no need for conversion to open surgery. Our recommendation is to keep the MIS approach, place as many external drains as necessary to avoid choleperitoneum or the accumulation of postoperative fluid collections and refer the patient to a specialized hepatobiliary surgery unit as soon as possible [4].

As regards the placement of external drains, the purpose is to leave the abdominal cavity clean and to direct the biliary fistula externally. Ideally, at least one of the

J. Goransky · G. Arbues (✉)
HPB Surgery, Hospital Italiano de San Justo, San Justo, Argentina
e-mail: guillermo.arbues@hospitalitaliano.org.ar

J. Pekolj et al. (eds.), *Fundamentals of Bile Duct Injuries*,
https://doi.org/10.1007/978-3-031-13383-1_14

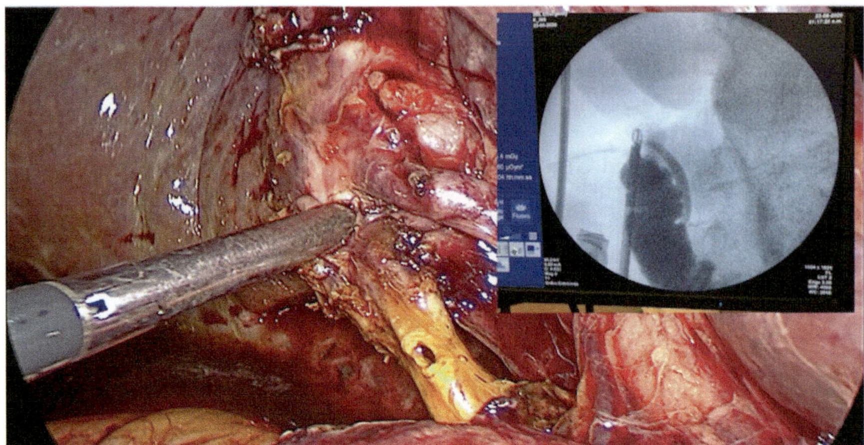

Fig. 14.1 Intraoperative diagnosis of a *Strasberg D* BDI by IOC

drains should be close to the site of the injury with the shortest possible distance to the skin.

Finally, and perhaps the most important thing to understand is that an open surgery only to confirm an obvious surgical injury and without immediate repair by an expert surgeon is not recommended. This decision may not only aggravate the injury due to less visibility and the stress of the situation, but it can also cause more adhesions that will make future treatments more challenging [5].

Treatment of the Choleperitoneum

If a BDI was not noticed during the primary surgery, the patient will present in the early postoperative period with abdominal and systemic manifestations *[See Chap. 8: Postoperative diagnosis of Bile Duct Injuries—The Surgeon's vision].*

Although it is very frequent to see patients with a BDI, whose bile leak had disseminated throughout the entire abdominal cavity causing *"choleperitoneum."*

If a patient in the early postoperative course of a cholecystectomy demonstrates signs of systemic inflammatory response syndrome (SIRS) along with abdominal compromise and radiographically evidence of free fluid, we should suspect choleperitoneum, and without question, a laparoscopic exploration should be guaranteed [6].

If the choleperitoneum is confirmed, thorough abdominal drainage and washout can be offered laparoscopically, in order to control and direct the bile leak externally.

MIS approaches facilitate the full exploration of the abdominal cavity, and the modern laparoscopic suction-irrigation systems permit an extensive washout.

In cases where more than 5 days have passed since the primary surgery, sometimes it is not possible to easily localize the site of the injury. In those cases, we do not recommend adamantly searching for the leaking site, since it may aggravate the injury or complicate it even more by adding an associated vascular injury (AVI) to this already unfortunate situation [7].

In the great majority of cases, completing an exhaustive abdominal washout and placing external drains suffice to contemporize the patient, externalize and prepare the definitive repair.

Role of MIS in the Definitive Treatment of a BDI

Depending on the patient's situation and the availability of a specialist, a definitive repair can be performed at two stages: ***intraoperatively*** or ***deferred*** after the patient has already been "contemporized."

Intraoperatively Recognized BDI

The definitive treatment of a BDI can occur either intraoperatively once the injury has been detected if the local conditions are favorable and the surgeon is sufficiently trained in MIS hepatobiliary surgery. Upfront repairs, whenever possible, provide the best long-term outcomes with minimal footprint on the patient [4, 8, 9] (Fig. 14.2).

However, the laparoscopic repair of BDI per se is closely related to the complexity of the injury. For Strasberg type A or D injuries that are recognized

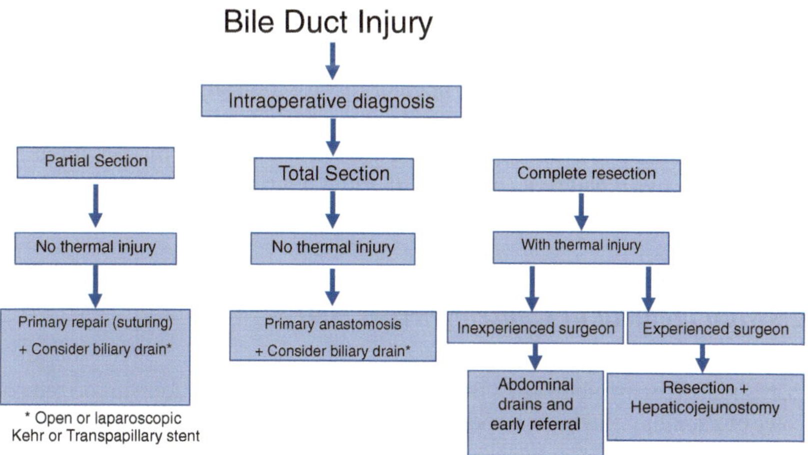

Fig. 14.2 Algorithm of intraoperative management of BDI

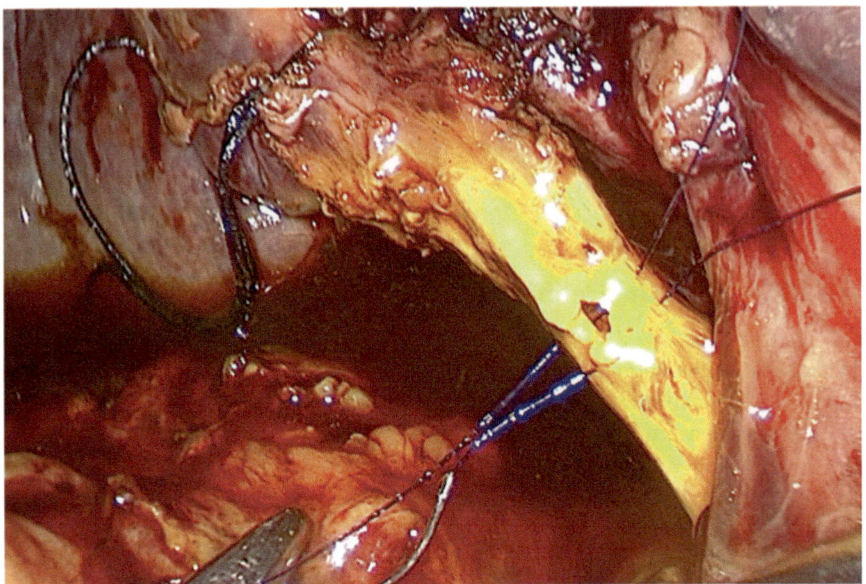

Fig. 14.3 *Strasberg D* BID treated laparoscopically by simple CBD primary closure with two interrupted 5-0 PDS

intraoperatively, or, at an early stage, they can be repaired using re-absorbable monofilament sutures in association with endoscopic support by means of ERCP (Fig. 14.3). Through this, either a clip can be placed/removed, or a suture can be made in combination with a *Distal Balloon Occlusion Cholangiogram*, with the eventual insertion of an *endobiliary prosthesis* [10].

In case of other types of lesions *(B, C, E),* depending on the patient's condition, the severity, and the physiopathology of injury, we have to analyze our two options consisting of:

- Immediate reconstruction (either open or laparoscopically) performed by a specialist [11].
- Insertion of external drains and contemporization until the local conditions facilitate a definitive repair (e.g., extensive thermal injury, an unpredictable extension of the injury in the acute phase, suspicion of an AVI) [12].

MIS Management of Contemporized BDI

Laparoscopic reconstruction of a BDI that has been previously contemporized could be very challenging and must be performed by a skilled and experienced surgeon [4] (Fig. 14.4).

Although the evidence for MIS biliary reconstruction after BDI is limited, there is vast experience using MIS approaches in the treatment of other benign (common

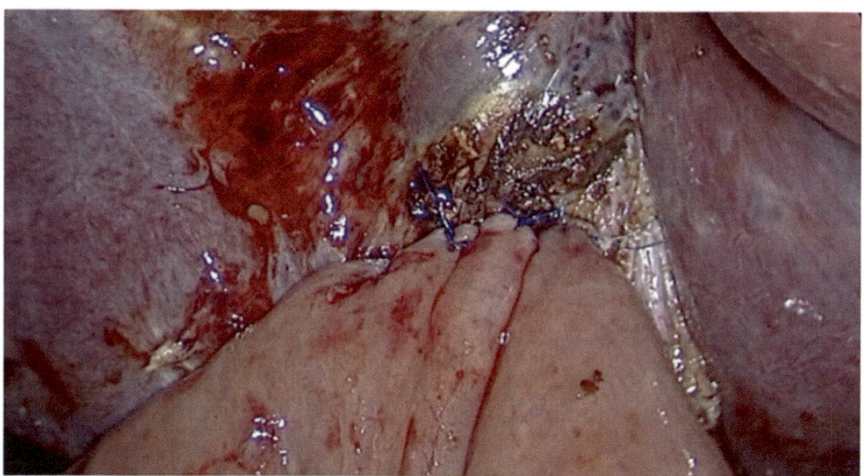

Fig. 14.4 *Strasberg E2* BID treated by laparoscopic Roux-en-Y HJ 8 weeks after the injury

bile duct cysts) and malignant (pancreatic cancer, cholangiocarcinoma) biliary pathologies where it has proven to be feasible and safe, with excellent long-term results [13–15].

There is also clear evidence that the best time to repair a BDI definitively is at an early stage (ideally before 72 h) or late (after 6 weeks) but never in between given the extensive locoregional inflammatory changes and remodellation that are present at that period of healing [16–18].

Likewise, besides the timing of repair, the success of long-term resolution is also related to proper eradication of any intra-abdominal infection, adequate nutritional status, complete cholangiogram, and the use of a proper technique for the reconstruction [8].

From a technical point of view, the essential aspects for a good short- and the long-term result after hepaticojejunostomy (HJ) have already been reported. The most important ones are a well-vascularized bile duct, tension-free anastomosis including the intestinal mucosa, with the largest possible diameter and complete biliary drainage of all hepatic segments [19] *[see Chap. 15: Biliodigestive anastomosis]*.

All these issues can be perfectly achieved with MIS, including better visibility on high-definition screens without the need for magnifying loupes, with proven benefits such as reduction in postoperative pain, blood loss, postoperative ileus, hospital stay, respiratory and cardiac complications, and finally better quality of life.

It is very important to have all adequate equipment ready for these cases, according to the SAGES guidelines for laparoscopic biliary surgery [20].

We personally recommend the use of fine laparoscopic needle drivers such as Jarit ® 600–249 curved tip since it makes a huge difference when manipulating such delicate tissues like the bile duct.

During the past years, with the advance in robotic surgery, experience with robotic HJ for BDIs has been published, nevertheless, in the unique paper that compared laparoscopic vs robotic biliary repair, there was no significant difference in any of the variables [21].

In conclusion, MIS approaches currently have a crucial role in the diagnosis and contemporization of a BDI, generating less systemic inflammatory response (accelerating recovery and externalization), fewer adherences for a definitive repair, and can be performed by a general surgeon with experience in laparoscopy [22].

Moreover, although the role of laparoscopy for a definitive repair of BDI is being increasingly accepted, it is still controversial, and it is recommended to be performed by an expert hepatobiliary surgeon [23].

References

1. Rystedt JML, Wiss J, Adolfsson J, Enochsson L, Hallerbäck B, Johansson P, et al. Routine versus selective intraoperative cholangiography during cholecystectomy: systematic review, meta-analysis, and health economic model analysis of iatrogenic bile duct injury. BJS Open [Internet]. 2021;5 https://doi.org/10.1093/bjsopen/zraa032.
2. Christou N, Roux-David A, Naumann DN, Bouvier S, Rivaille T, Derbal S, et al. Bile duct injury during cholecystectomy: necessity to learn how to do and interpret intraoperative cholangiography. Front Med. 2021;8:637987.
3. Alvarez FA, de Santibañes M, Palavecino M, Sánchez Clariá R, Mazza O, Arbues G, et al. Impact of routine intraoperative cholangiography during laparoscopic cholecystectomy on bile duct injury. Br J Surg. 2014;101:677–84.
4. El Nakeeb A, Sultan A, Ezzat H, Attia M, Abd ElWahab M, Kayed T, et al. Impact of referral pattern and timing of repair on surgical outcome after reconstruction of post-cholecystectomy bile duct injury: a multicenter study. Hepatobiliary Pancreat Dis Int. 2021;20:53–60.
5. de'Angelis N, Catena F, Memeo R, Coccolini F, Martínez-Pérez A, Romeo OM, et al. WSES guidelines for the detection and management of bile duct injury during cholecystectomy. World J Emerg Surg. 2020;2021(16):30.
6. Kaukonen K-M, Bailey M, Pilcher D, Cooper DJ, Bellomo R. Systemic inflammatory response syndrome criteria in defining severe sepsis. N Engl J Med. 2015;372:1629–38.
7. Schmidt SC, Settmacher U, Langrehr JM, Neuhaus P. Management and outcome of patients with combined bile duct and hepatic arterial injuries after laparoscopic cholecystectomy. Surgery. 2004;135:613–8.
8. Pekolj J, Alvarez FA, Palavecino M, Sánchez Clariá R, Mazza O, de Santibañes E. Intraoperative management and repair of bile duct injuries sustained during 10,123 laparoscopic cholecystectomies in a high-volume referral center. J Am Coll Surg. 2013;216:894–901.
9. Lau WY, Lai ECH, Lau SHY. Management of bile duct injury after laparoscopic cholecystectomy: a review. ANZ J Surg. 2010;80:75–81.
10. Katsinelos P, Kountouras J, Paroutoglou G, Beltsis A, Zavos C, Chatzimavroudis G, et al. The role of endoscopic treatment in postoperative bile leaks. Hepato-Gastroenterology. 2006;53:166–70.
11. Cuendis-Velázquez A, Morales-Chávez C, Aguirre-Olmedo I, Torres-Ruiz F, Rojano-Rodríguez M, Fernández-Álvarez L, et al. Laparoscopic hepaticojejunostomy after bile duct injury. Surg Endosc. 2016;30:876–82.

12. Pekolj J, Drago J. Controversies in iatrogenic bile duct injuries. Role of video-assisted laparoscopy in the management of iatrogenic bile duct injuries. Cir Esp. 2020;98:61–3.
13. Liem NT, Pham HD, Dung LA, Son TN, Vu HM. Early and intermediate outcomes of laparoscopic surgery for choledochal cysts with 400 patients. J Laparoendosc Adv Surg Tech A. 2012;22:599–603.
14. Shen H-J, Xu M, Zhu H-Y, Yang C, Li F, Li K-W, et al. Laparoscopic versus open surgery in children with choledochal cysts: a meta-analysis. Pediatr Surg Int. 2015;31:529–34.
15. Rahnemai-Azar AA, Abbasi A, Tsilimigras DI, Weber SM, Pawlik TM. Current advances in minimally invasive surgical management of perihilar cholangiocarcinoma. J Gastrointest Surg. 2020;24:2143–9.
16. Iannelli A, Paineau J, Hamy A, Schneck A-S, Schaaf C, Gugenheim J. Primary versus delayed repair for bile duct injuries sustained during cholecystectomy: results of a survey of the Association Francaise de Chirurgie. HPB. 2013;15:611–6.
17. Schreuder AM, Nunez Vas BC, Booij KAC, van Dieren S, Besselink MG, Busch OR, et al. Optimal timing for surgical reconstruction of bile duct injury: meta-analysis. BJS Open. 2020;4:776–86.
18. Karanikas M, Bozali F, Vamvakerou V, Markou M, Memet Chasan ZT, Efraimidou E, et al. Biliary tract injuries after lap cholecystectomy-types, surgical intervention and timing. Ann Transl Med. 2016;4:163.
19. Stewart L, Way LW. Bile duct injuries during laparoscopic cholecystectomy. Factors that influence the results of treatment. Arch Surg. 1995;130:1123–8. discussion 1129
20. Scott-Conner CEH, editor. The SAGES manual: fundamentals of laparoscopy, thoracoscopy, and GI endoscopy. New York, NY: Springer; 2006.
21. Cuendis-Velázquez A, Trejo-Ávila M, Bada-Yllán O, Cárdenas-Lailson E, Morales-Chávez C, Fernández-Álvarez L, et al. A new era of bile duct repair: robotic-assisted versus laparoscopic hepaticojejunostomy. J Gastrointest Surg. 2019;23:451–9.
22. Overby DW, Apelgren KN, Richardson W, Fanelli R. Society of American Gastrointestinal and Endoscopic Surgeons. SAGES guidelines for the clinical application of laparoscopic biliary tract surgery. Surg Endosc. 2010;24:2368–86.
23. Drago J, de Santibañes M, Palavecino M, Sánchez Clariá R, Arbues G, Mazza O, Pekolj J. Role of laparoscopy in the immediate, intermediate, and long-term management of iatrogenic bile duct injuries during laparoscopic cholecystectomy. Langenbecks Arch Surg. 2022;407(2):663–73.

Chapter 15
Biliodigestive Anastomosis

David Alberto Biagiola, Juan Glinka, and Rodrigo Sánchez Claria

Introduction

Biliodigestive Anastomosis (BA) is the first surgical option for the primary reconstruction BDI and in those where primary repairs or non-operative (endoscopic, percutaneous) treatments were not successful [1].

There are multiple variables that influence the outcome of a BA in the context of a BDI that a surgeon must consider. The level, extension, and degree of vascular involvement of the injury will determine the type of BA that would be better applicable for certain patients.

Moreover, *odds for a successful repair are proportionally inverse to the height of the injury.* That is to say, the higher the injuries the more technically challenging the reconstruction will be, as they have a greater likelihood of ischemic compromise and increased chances of long-term strictures [2].

In addition, when the injury is high enough to require a BA between two or more separate ducts, the reconstruction is even more challenging, and therefore the risk of failure is also higher [3].

In addition, the presence of secondary biliary cirrhosis (CBS) with or without portal hypertension (PHT) is an extremely important aspect to look for, when

D. A. Biagiola
HPB Surgery and Liver Transplant Unit, Sanatorio Parque, Rosario, Argentina

J. Glinka
Division of HPB Surgery and Multiorgan Transplant Unit, Western University – London Regional Cancer Program, London, ON, Canada

R. Sánchez Claria (✉)
HPB Surgery and Intestinal Transplant Unit, Hospital Italiano de Buenos Aires, Buenos Aires, Argentina
e-mail: rodrigo.sanchez@hospitalitaliano.org.ar

J. Pekolj et al. (eds.), *Fundamentals of Bile Duct Injuries*,
https://doi.org/10.1007/978-3-031-13383-1_15

planning a biliary reconstruction. Although these patients can be completely asymptomatic from a liver perspective, reconstruction in the context of cirrhosis is set to fail. Any suspicion of it should set off a FibroScan or even better a liver biopsy, and if positive for fibrosis, referral for liver transplant center for assessment should be arranged immediately [4].

The presence of associated vascular injury (AVI) is a crucial prognostic factor. All the patients planned for a reconstruction following a BDI must undergo at least a CT angiography for vascular assessment of the liver and celiac trunk. If there is any doubt or uncertainty, a conventional angiography should be arranged given that AVI is very frequent (up to 25% of complex BDI) and determine the outcome of further therapies [5] *[See Chap. 10 Assessment of vascular structures in Bile Duct Injuries].*

Special Considerations

There are different types of BA that are used with different indications. However, the *Roux-en-Y hepaticojejunostomy (RYHJ)* is always the first choice in the context of BDIs.

The *choledocho-duodenal anastomosis* (CDA) would not be our first alternative, given that it does not exclude the biliary tree from the alimentary transit, having greater incidence of cholangitis, and most importantly, higher incidence of cholangiocarcinoma in the long run. This is particularly concerning in young patients with a reasonable life expectancy, as demonstrated in numerous series.

Patients with BDI have received multiple previous therapies such as conversion to open surgery, reoperations for bile leaks, bleedings, previous repair attempts, percutaneous drains, ERCP with stenting, etc. Consequently, it is not unfrequent to have a frozen porta hepatis (PH) as a result of multiple inflammatory adhesions at different stages of remodelation.

Moreover, when there is an AVI, the phenomenon of atrophy-hypertrophy of the injured-healthy lobe can distort the anatomy even more. Therefore, the recognition of the structures within the PH can be challenging for even the most experienced surgeons.

In such complicated scenarios, the IOC is a great ally. This could be accomplished through different strategies, either by puncturing the CBD above the stricture, palpating the biliary stent if any, or performing a cholangiogram through a PBD if this is in place.

It also provides a mapping of the intrahepatic biliary tree to ensure that all the segments are connected and adequately drained, and also confirms that the site we have chosen for the anastomosis is above the stricture.

The role of indocyanine green (ICG) seems to be very promising to help identify the anatomy, although there is no validation of its application for this situation.

Technique

Once we delineate the anastomotic site on the bile duct, the inframesocolic compartment of the abdomen is then accessed to identify the angle of Treitz and the first fixed intestinal loop. From this point, the second or third jejunal loop is selected to find the one that reaches the PH free of tension, and preferentially in an isoperistaltic fashion [6]. The jejunum is then divided at this level, and a hand-sewn or stapled jejunal-jejunal (JJ) anastomosis is made leaving at least 60–70 cm of length, in order to keep it completely defunctionalized from the digestive tract to prevent recurrent cholangitis.

Finally, we ascend the jejunal loop via the transmesocolic route with the candy cane anatomically directed towards the left.

These steps are standard for any type of Roux-en-Y HJ. Next, we will analyze three considerations for creating the BD, depending on the *height* of the BDI according to the *Bismuth–Corlette classification.*

In **Bismuth type I** injuries, an end-to-side HJ is performed. If the bile duct is larger than 6 mm, the posterior wall can be performed in a continuous fashion using preferentially a reabsorbable suture like 5-0/6-0 Polydioxanone. The anterior wall can be reconstructed with the same sutures in an interrupted fashion. If *it is smaller than 6 mm, interrupted suturing using Polydioxanone, or 7-0 Polypropylene is usually recommended.* However, the fact that *non-absorbable sutures could be lithogenic in the long run* has to be kept in mind (Fig. 15.1).

In **Bismuth type II** injuries, a wide opening of the left hepatic duct can be made, as described by Hepp and Couinaud. In this type of BA, the opening is usually wide, so we use 5-0 or 6-0 threads of the above-mentioned material, in either a continuous

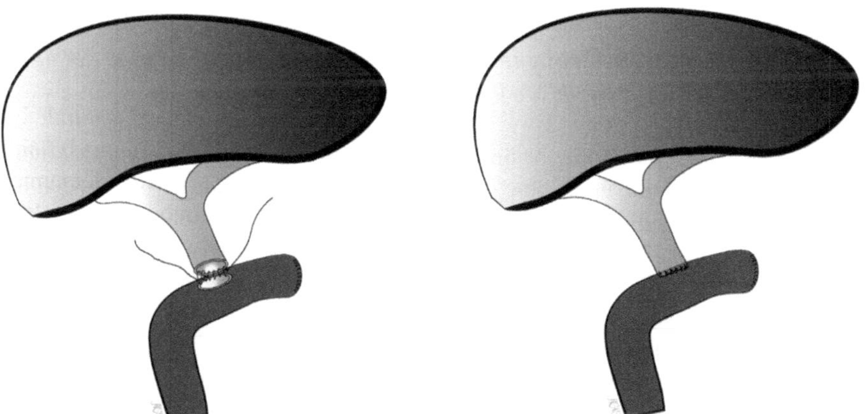

Fig. 15.1 Biliary reconstruction in Bismuth type I injuries end to side Roux-en-Y Hepaticojejunostomy

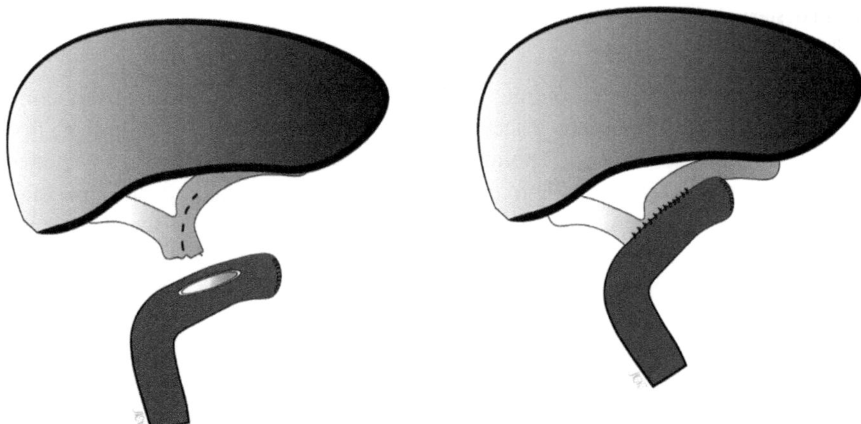

Fig. 15.2 Example of Hepp–Couinaud biliary reconstruction

or interrupted fashion for the anterior wall. The CBD distal to the stricture can be either preserved (lateral-lateral reconstruction) or resected [7, 8] (Fig. 15.2).

In **Bismuth type III** and **Bismuth type IV** injuries, the reconstruction is frequently complex and technically demanding. The hepatic ducts must be accessed separately above the injury. The dissection planes are challenging since it is required to navigate between the already fibrotic hilar plate and inflammatory planes around the injury [9]. On occasions, an hepatotomy at the base of segment IVb may be required to have better access to the suprahilar structures (hepatic ducts).

Reconstruction of Multiple Ducts

If there are several ducts, *trying to reconstruct them together in order to obtain as few anastomoses as possible would be recommended*, although this is not always possible [10, 11].

In cases in which multiple reconstructions are required, the recommended technique is to perform the entire row of posterior walls first, followed by the anterior wall, instead of completing one anastomosis after the other as usual [12].

To achieve this, interrupted sutures are placed on the anterior wall of the different ducts. These sutures will hold the anterior walls open, facilitating the back wall optimal visualization and thus the suture placement there. Next, the first enterotomy of the jejunum will be made followed by placing the *stay sutures* on the corners. The sutures of the posterior wall are then placed inside-out on the jejunum and outside-in on the hepatic duct. The other enterotomies are created and interrupted sutures are placed on the posterior wall of all multiple ducts as well. Afterward, all posterior wall sutures are placed, before tying the stitches to maintain a clear view for suture placements. We have to be certain that the

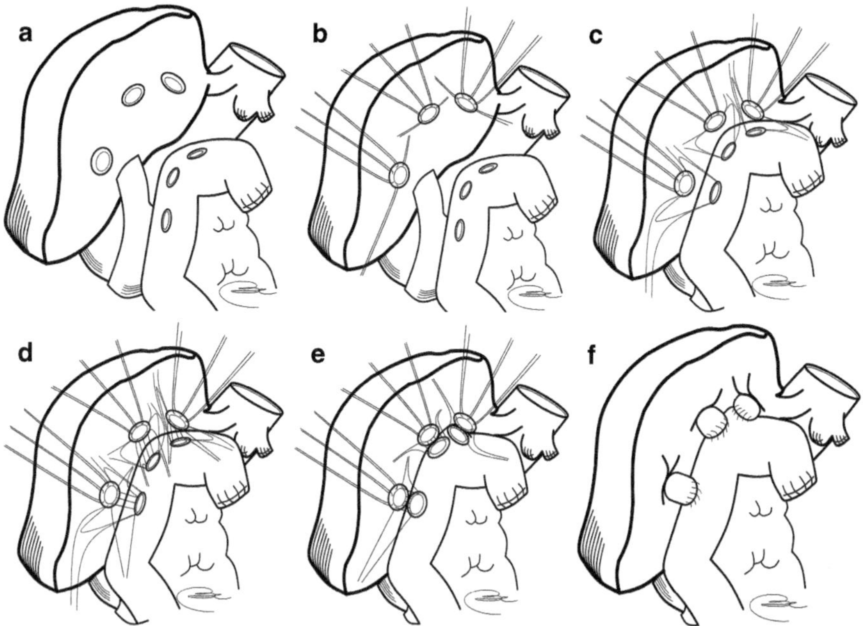

Fig. 15.3 Sequence when multiple separate biliary ducts need to be reconstructed. (**a**) The hepatic ducts and the jejunum Roux-en-Y loop are represented. (**b**) Stitches that will hold the anterior walls of the different ducts open, facilitating the back wall optimal visualization and thus the suture placement are placed in an interrupted fashion. (**c**) "*Stay sutures*" are placed on the corners. (**d**) Interrupted sutures on the *posterior wall* of the different ducts are then placed inside-out on the jejunum and outside-in on the hepatic ducts. (**e**) The posterior wall stitches are tied (knots inside). (**f**) The anterior wall stitches are tied and the anastomosis is concluded (knots outside)

distance between each enterotomy is in accordance with the distance between the ducts to ensure reconstruction is free of tension.

Subsequently, the jejunum is parachuted down to the duct orifices and the posterior wall sutures are tied on the inside. The anterior row of sutures will next be placed on the jejunum and complete the anastomosis with knots tied on the outside.

The thickness of the suture thread will depend on the caliber and quality of the bile duct wall; however, resorbable material (preferably Polydioxanone) is recommended here especially as the posterior wall knots remain on the inside (of the anastomosis).

Particular attention has to be paid to the thread management, having the sutures organized and preventing entanglement with the help of numerous "rubber-shod clamps." It is mandatory to perform the different anastomosis in an interrupted fashion, in order to minimize not only ischemia but also centripetal traction of a continuous suture over the lumen of the small bile duct, which may facilitate anastomotic stenosis (Fig. 15.3a–f).

We do not usually calibrate the anastomosis with internal or external catheters or stents.

In the presence of very high bile duct injuries, in which second-order ducts are involved, it is recommended to perform a hepatic resection and make an HJ to the contralateral hepatic duct [13, 14].

Frequent Complications of Biliodigestive Anastomosis

Bile Leak Most observed in the early postoperative period. It is frequently a consequence of an inadequate technique or secondary to partial dehiscence of the BA secondary to ischemia of the distal end of the bile duct. This complication is more frequent in patients with high-level bile duct resections such as those performed due to Klatskin tumors, and when anastomosis of multiple ducts is required.

As the dehiscences of an RYHJ are usually partial and naturally excluded from the intestinal transit, they are self-limited. Their treatment though, will vary according to the clinical condition from mini-invasive endoscopic or percutaneous drainage to operation and redo of the HJ whenever possible [15, 16].

Cholangitis This is usually associated with some degree of obstruction to the bile outflow, although not only at the level of the anastomosis. Matthews et al. monitored 24 patients with recurrent cholangitis in BA that up to 35% of the cases there was no anastomotic stricture, rather than associated factors such as another intrahepatic stricture secondary to excluded ducts, inadequate construction of the anastomotic loop, and conditions that predispose to bacterial overgrowth like a *blind loop syndrome* secondary to a long candy cane [17, 18].

Non-obstructive afferent loop syndrome can be caused by any degree of distal obstruction either from the jejuno-jejunostomy or from any portion of the distal bowel secondary to postoperative adhesions, etc. [19].

The *Sump Syndrome* is also caused by non-obstructive reflux of gastrointestinal content into the biliary tree causing usually mild recurrent episodes of cholangitis. It must be considered when other causes including strictures have been ruled out. These patients are usually treated with prophylactic antibiotic therapy [18, 20].

The importance of recurrent cholangitis in these patients lies in the acute septic complications, the deterioration of liver function conditioning progressive fibrosis factor, and the development of SBC. It is extremely important to map the biliary tree before a reconstruction, to be sure all of the above is addressed beforehand.

Cholangiocarcinoma The chronic inflammation within the biliary tree has been associated with the development of bile duct tumors. In a study by Tocchi et al. in the long-term follow-up of 1003 patients who underwent BA for benign non-neoplastic pathology, biliary tumors occurred in 55 patients, corresponding to 5.5% of the population. In that series, it occurred between 11 and 19 years after surgery and was more frequent in CDA (7.6%) than in transduodenal papillotomy (5.8%) or RYHJ (1.9%) [21].

Interestingly, *recurrent cholangitis was present in 72%* of cases that developed tumors, which were also more frequent in cases with Oddi disease (7.2%) than in cases of lithiasis (5.9%) or postoperative stricture (1.9%) [22].

The prognosis of these patients was discouraging, as 34 patients were considered inoperable, 9 received an exploratory laparotomy with an intraoperative diagnosis of unresectability and only 12 were resected with curative intention. Nevertheless, all of them died within 9 months after resection [21].

Strictures This is the *most frequent* late complication that if left untreated can have irreversible sequelae and consequences.

Its occurrence was classically described to be between 5% and 15% of cases in the open surgery era (45% within the first 2 years and 80% within 5 years). However, in the laparoscopic era, stricture rates post-reconstruction are higher and earlier because the mechanism of injury is different (higher and usually thermal injuries).

Schol et al. reported an incidence of 26% of anastomotic strictures, being earlier (average 138 days) and more frequent in higher repairs (Bismuth III and IV) [23].

Interestingly, they observed that when the repair was deferred, (more than 6–8 weeks), the long-term results were adequate in 94% of the cases treated by the same team, concluding that an early repair over damaged and ischemic tissues represents an important factor in the genesis of stricture.

The diagnosis of stenosis is clinically evidenced by episodes of cholangitis, abdominal pain, or jaundice. However, a period of asymptomatic evolution is frequent and should be considered in the follow-up of the patient by laboratory and imaging tests.

Follow-Up

After a BA, periodic monitoring of the serum alkaline phosphatase (ALP) levels should be part of the basic "screening" for any patient with any kind of BA reconstruction.

ALP can be elevated even before the bilirubin levels rise, indicating incipient cholestasis.

Although the majority of these patients have naturally higher ALP levels, generally do not exceed twice the normal limits [24].

It is important then to observe its trend over time, and if it continues to rise over time, ruling out the presence of stricture with more accurate methods becomes mandatory.

We resumed in Table 15.1, Schweizer et al. proposal for the assessment of the outcomes following an RYHJ [25].

Sometimes we can have cholestasis and still have normal caliber bile ducts in a routine ultrasound (US). Magnetic resonance cholangiopancreatography (MRCP) is used as a non-invasive method to confirm this, having a certainty rate of 93% in the diagnosis of even subtle anastomotic strictures. In uncertain cases, functional

Table 15.1 Outcomes assessment following a Roux-en-Y Hepaticojejunostomy

Outcome	Symptoms	Alkaline phosphatase	Imaging workup
Excellent	Absent	Normal	No obstruction or lithiasis
Good	Absent	High	No obstruction or lithiasis
Regular	Improvement	High	Evidence of obstruction and/or lithiasis
Bad	Persistent or worsening	High	Evidence of obstruction and/or lithiasis

studies like hepatobiliary scintigraphy (HIDA) scan have been extremely useful, as it can reveal segmental or unilateral stenosis due to the retention of the isotopic marker in a determined sector of the liver [26–28].

Finally, percutaneous transhepatic cholangiography (PTC) is an excellent study that allows the precise delimitation of the biliary tree and it permits the placement of a percutaneous biliary drainage (PBD) in the same procedure to consequently arrange dilatations if a stricture is encountered [29].

If none of these methods observe any cause of cholestasis, it is mandatory to exclude hepatocellular causes for it like fibrosis or ongoing cirrhosis among others [30].

Treatment of Post BA Strictures

Once a stricture of the anastomosis is confirmed, the treatment depends on the type of anastomosis, the general condition of the patient, the height of the injury, and the experience of the treating team [21].

If the stenosis is located in a choledocho-duodenal anastomosis, the initial treatment should be endoscopic, considering balloon dilatation. However, converting this reconstruction to an HJ should be highly considered in patients with a good life expectancy for the aforementioned reasons.

In the case of stenosis of the RYHJ, the percutaneous approach is in general the first option. It also facilitates dilatation. There are several percutaneous protocols of successive dilatations that can be implemented [31, 32].

However, if this remains to be ineffective, a redo HJ is highly effective (>90%) when performed by trained groups in this type of complex surgery, as shown in several recent series [13, 33].

In complex injuries with predictable failure rates, it should also be considered to perform a *Hutson-Russel loop*. This essentially consists of securing an intestinal loop (in continuity to the BA) into the anterior abdominal wall and marking it with a radiopaque marker. As a result, this loop can be easily accessed percutaneously and facilitates transjejunal procedures including dilatations [34].

Quality of life (QoL) should be considered in scenarios like this that could require numerous and successive procedures. Accordingly, Boerma and Melton demonstrated in their respective publications, less invasive but repeated procedures have not produced exceedingly better results on QoL compared to upfront surgical treatment. Therefore, for patients who do not desire repeated dilation and are considered good surgical candidates, we recommend upfront surgical reconstruction [35, 36].

Prevention of the stricture after an RYHJ is key. To achieve this, maximizing outcomes during the reconstruction, where a tension-free, mucosa–mucosa apposition on healthy and well-irrigated tissues is mandatory. Moreover, the use of fine (6-0/7-0) absorbable sutures along with magnification is extremely important as well [5].

The minimally invasive approach is not considered the standard of care at present, although an increasing number of publications have emerged in recent years, in which selected successful cases of laparoscopic repairs have been reported [37–39].

References

1. Asbun HJ, Rossi RL, Lowell JA, Munson JL. Bile duct injury during laparoscopic cholecystectomy: mechanism of injury, prevention, and management. World J Surg. 1993;17:547–51. 551–2
2. Misra S, Melton GB, Geschwind JF, Venbrux AC, Cameron JL, Lillemoe KD. Percutaneous management of bile duct strictures and injuries associated with laparoscopic cholecystectomy: a decade of experience. J Am Coll Surg. 2004;198:218–26.
3. Mercado MA, Chan C, Orozco H, Tielve M, Hinojosa CA. Acute bile duct injury. The need for a high repair. Surg Endosc. 2003;17:1351–5.
4. Sulpice L, Garnier S, Rayar M, Meunier B, Boudjema K. Biliary cirrhosis and sepsis are two risk factors of failure after surgical repair of major bile duct injury post-laparoscopic cholecystectomy. Langenbeck's Arch Surg. 2014;399:601–8.
5. De Santibáñes E, Ardiles V, Pekolj J. Complex bile duct injuries: management. HPB. 2008;10:4–12.
6. Zorn GL 3rd, Wright JK, Pinson CW, Debelak JP, Chapman WC. Antiperistaltic Roux-en-Y biliary-enteric bypass after bile duct injury: a technical error in reconstruction. Am Surg. 1999;65:581–5.
7. Myburgh JA. The Hepp-Couinaud approach to strictures of the bile ducts. I. Injuries, choledochal cysts, and pancreatitis. Ann Surg. 1993;218:615–20.
8. Hepp J. Hepaticojejunostomy using the left biliary trunk for iatrogenic biliary lesions: the French connection. World J Surg. 1985;9:507–11.
9. Strasberg SM, Picus DD, Drebin JA. Results of a new strategy for reconstruction of biliary injuries having an isolated right-sided component. J Gastrointest Surg. 2001;5:266–74.
10. Salvalaggio PRO, Whitington PF, Alonso EM, Superina RA. Presence of multiple bile ducts in the liver graft increases the incidence of biliary complications in pediatric liver transplantation. Liver Transpl. 2005;11:161–6.
11. Chok KSH, Lo CM. Systematic review and meta-analysis of studies of biliary reconstruction in adult living donor liver transplantation. ANZ J Surg. 2017;87:121–5.
12. Hirano S, Tanaka E, Tsuchikawa T, Matsumoto J, Shichinohe T, Kato K. Techniques of biliary reconstruction following bile duct resection (with video). J Hepatobiliary Pancreat Sci. 2012;19:203–9.
13. Benkabbou A, Castaing D, Salloum C, Adam R, Azoulay D, Vibert E. Treatment of failed Roux-en-Y hepaticojejunostomy after post-cholecystectomy bile ducts injuries. Surgery. 2013;153:95–102.

14. Li J, Frilling A, Nadalin S, Broelsch CE, Malago M. Timing and risk factors of hepatectomy in the management of complications following laparoscopic cholecystectomy. J Gastrointest Surg. 2012;16:815–20.
15. Luigiano C, Iabichino G, Mangiavillano B, et al. Endoscopic management of bile duct injury after hepatobiliary tract surgery: a comprehensive review. Minerva Chir. 2016;71:398–406.
16. Vidovszky AA, Qafiti F, El Haddi SJ, Doukides T, Hus N, Genuit T. The use of percutaneous-endoscopic rendezvous stenting in a patient with bile duct injury after cholecystectomy—and a unique complication requiring secondary endoscopic intervention. J Surg Case Rep. 2021;2021:rjab119.
17. Carrel T, Matthews J, Schweizer W, Baer H, Gertsch P, Blumgart LH. Diagnosis, etiology and treatment of cholangitis following bilio-digestive surgery. Helv Chir Acta. 1990;56:891–6.
18. Matthews JB, Baer HU, Schweizer WP, Gertsch P, Carrel T, Blumgart LH. Recurrent cholangitis with and without anastomotic stricture after biliary-enteric bypass. Arch Surg. 1993;128:269–72.
19. Sanada Y, Yamada N, Taguchi M, et al. Recurrent cholangitis by biliary stasis due to non-obstructive afferent loop syndrome after pylorus-preserving pancreatoduodenectomy: report of a case. Int Surg. 2014;99:426–31.
20. Marangoni G, Ali A, Faraj W, Heaton N, Rela M. Clinical features and treatment of sump syndrome following hepaticojejunostomy. Hepatobiliary Pancreat Dis Int. 2011;10:261–4.
21. Tocchi A, Mazzoni G, Liotta G, Lepre L, Cassini D, Miccini M. Late development of bile duct cancer in patients who had biliary-enteric drainage for benign disease: a follow-up study of more than 1,000 patients. Ann Surg. 2001;234:210–4.
22. Ma KW, Cheung TT, She WH, Chok KSH, Yan Chan AC, Chiu Dai JW, Lo CM. Recurrent pyogenic cholangitis - an independent poor prognostic indicator for resectable intrahepatic cholangiocarcinoma: a propensity score matched analysis. HPB. 2018;20:1067–72.
23. Schol FP, Go PM, Gouma DJ. Risk factors for bile duct injury in laparoscopic cholecystectomy: analysis of 49 cases. Br J Surg. 1994;81:1786–8.
24. Negi SS, Chaudhary A. Analysis of abnormal recovery pattern of liver function tests after surgical repair of bile duct strictures. J Gastroenterol Hepatol. 2005;20:1533–7.
25. Zielsdorf SM, Klein JJ, Fleetwood VA, Hertl M, Chan EY. Hepaticojejunostomy for benign disease: long-term stricture rate and management. Am Surg. 2019;85:1350–3.
26. Sharma P, Kumar R, Das KJ, Singh H, Pal S, Parshad R, Bal C, Bandopadhyaya GP, Malhotra A. Detection and localization of post-operative and post-traumatic bile leak: hybrid SPECT-CT with 99mTc-Mebrofenin. Abdom Imaging. 2012;37:803–11.
27. Hyodo T, Kumano S, Kushihata F, Okada M, Hirata M, Tsuda T, Takada Y, Mochizuki T, Murakami T. CT and MR cholangiography: advantages and pitfalls in perioperative evaluation of biliary tree. Br J Radiol. 2012;85:887–96.
28. Suthar M, Purohit S, Bhargav V, Goyal P. Role of MRCP in differentiation of benign and malignant causes of biliary obstruction. J Clin Diagn Res. 2015;9:TC08–12.
29. Thompson CM, Saad NE, Quazi RR, Darcy MD, Picus DD, Menias CO. Management of iatrogenic bile duct injuries: role of the interventional radiologist. Radiographics. 2013;33:117–34.
30. AbdelRafee A, El-Shobari M, Askar W, Sultan AM, El Nakeeb A. Long-term follow-up of 120 patients after hepaticojejunostomy for treatment of post-cholecystectomy bile duct injuries: a retrospective cohort study. Int J Surg. 2015;18:205–10.
31. Czerwonko ME, Huespe P, Mazza O, de Santibanes M, Sanchez-Claria R, Pekolj J, Ciardullo M, de Santibanes E, Hyon SH. Percutaneous biliary balloon dilation: impact of an institutional three-session protocol on patients with benign anastomotic strictures of Hepatojejunostomy. Dig Surg. 2018;35:397–405.
32. Bang Y, Patil S, Singh J, Rabella P, Rao GV. Percutaneous biliary balloon dilatation and sequential upsizing of silastic transanastomotic stents for benign hepaticojejunostomy strictures: long-term results. HPB. 2018;20:S747.
33. Walsh RM, Matthew Walsh R, Michael Henderson J, Vogt DP, Brown N. Long-term outcome of biliary reconstruction for bile duct injuries from laparoscopic cholecystectomies. Surgery. 2007;142:450–7.

34. Riaz A, Entezari P, Ganger D, et al. Percutaneous access of the modified Hutson loop for retrograde cholangiography, endoscopy, and biliary interventions. J Vasc Interv Radiol. 2020;31:2113–2120.e1.
35. Pitt HA, Kaufman SL, Coleman J, White RI, Cameron JL. Benign postoperative biliary strictures. Operate or dilate? Ann Surg. 1989;210:417–25. discussion 426–7
36. Booij KAC, de Reuver PR, van Dieren S, van Delden OM, Rauws EA, Busch OR, van Gulik TM, Gouma DJ. Long-term impact of bile duct injury on morbidity, mortality, quality of life, and work related limitations. Ann Surg. 2018;268:143–50.
37. Cuendis-Velázquez A, Morales-Chávez C, Aguirre-Olmedo I, Torres-Ruiz F, Rojano-Rodríguez M, Fernández-Álvarez L, Cárdenas-Lailson E, Moreno-Portillo M. Laparoscopic hepaticojejunostomy after bile duct injury. Surg Endosc. 2016;30:876–82.
38. Cuendis-Velázquez A, Trejo-Ávila M, Bada-Yllán O, Cárdenas-Lailson E, Morales-Chávez C, Fernández-Álvarez L, Romero-Loera S, Rojano-Rodríguez M, Valenzuela-Salazar C, Moreno-Portillo M. A new era of bile duct repair: robotic-assisted versus laparoscopic hepaticojejunostomy. J Gastrointest Surg. 2019;23:451–9.
39. Drago J, de Santibañes M, Palavecino M, Sánchez Clariá R, Arbues G, Mazza O, Pekolj J. Role of laparoscopy in the immediate, intermediate, and long-term management of iatrogenic bile duct injuries during laparoscopic cholecystectomy. Langenbecks Arch Surg. 2022;407(2):663–73.

Chapter 16
Liver Resections

Julio César Lazarte and Juan Pekolj

Introduction

In the era of open cholecystectomy, a liver resection (LR) for the definitive treatment of a BDI has been an exceptional indication [1]. However, the laparoscopic approach introduced different mechanisms of injury that started to play a role. In consequence, it is more common to see higher, thermally induced BDIs, and/or *Associated with Vascular Injuries (AVI)* [2]. As a result, about 5–10% of patients with a BDI will require a LR for definitive management according to recent data [3].

Practically, the indications of a LR can be analyzed from two different perspectives.

BDI with AVI

Isolated injuries to the right hepatic artery (RHA) are generally well tolerated. In fact, an autopsy series demonstrated 7% of RHA injury in cadavers with a history of open cholecystectomy that died of a different cause and never had clinical manifestations of the arterial injury whatsoever [4]. To understand this, and the impact of the AVI in the management and prognosis of patients with BDIs it is key to review the role of the *hilar plexus (HP)* [5] (Fig. 16.1).

J. C. Lazarte
HPB Surgery, Clínica Pasteur, Neuquen, Argentina

J. Pekolj (✉)
General Surgery Service & Liver, Transplant Unit, Buenos Aires, Buenos Aires, Argentina
e-mail: juan.pekolj@hospitalitaliano.org.ar

J. Pekolj et al. (eds.), *Fundamentals of Bile Duct Injuries*,
https://doi.org/10.1007/978-3-031-13383-1_16

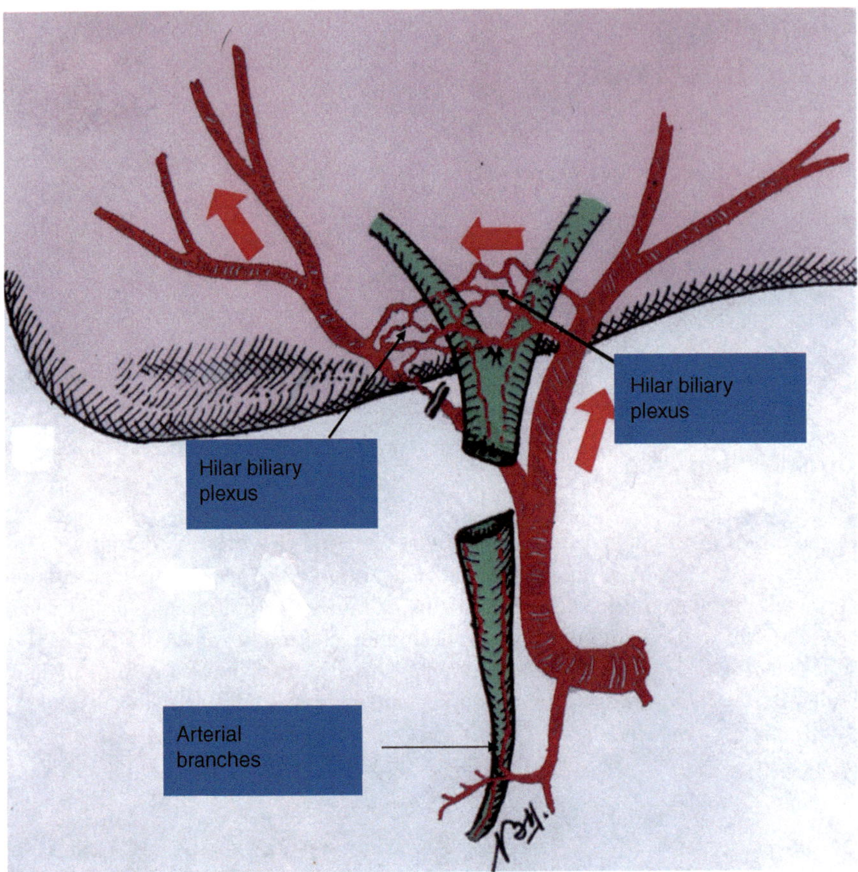

Fig. 16.1 Schematic picture of the hilar plexus provides collateralization between the right and left hepatic artery and is able to compensate for the loss of arterial inflow if one of these main branches is affected

The HP vascular network provides collateralization between the RHA and the left hepatic artery (LHA) and can compensate for the loss of arterial inflow if one of these main hepatic arteries (HA) branches is affected. It also represents the main arterial blood supply to the biliary confluence (BC) [6] (Fig. 16.2a, b).

That is to say, when a BDI is associated with a lesion of the RHA lets the left hepatic duct (LHD) well vascularized by the branches from the LHA and especially the segmental branch of sector IV. However, it also leaves the right hepatic duct (RHD) only irrigated by the HP [7]. This accessory route can be *primarily* compromised in *Strasberg type E4* injuries, as the BC is involved along with the AVI to the RHA, both the longitudinal shunt of the marginals and the transverse HP will be affected, shutting down the compensatory flow to the right hemiliver [6, 8, 9].

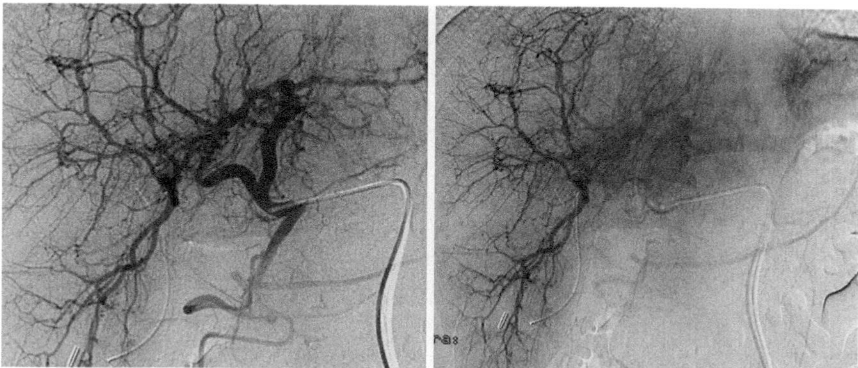

Fig. 16.2 Digital angiography in a patient with an injury in the right hepatic artery, receiving arterial supply from the left through a greatly developed hilar plexus

Consequently, the right lobe will have a high risk of ischemia and intrahepatic ischemic cholangiopathy (IC). *The higher the lesion, the more likely it is to affect the compensatory system of the HP and ultimately affect the arterial supply to the liver with their respective consequences, especially on the biliary tree* [10].

The HP can be injured *secondarily* as well during high biliary repairs and lead to the development of an early failure of the attempted reconstruction (Fig. 16.3a–d).

BDI with AVI is remarkably frequent (27–61% of overall BDIs) and implies a highly complex condition in which the outcome of the biliary repairs and the subsequent evolution of the patient are uncertain [11].

Therefore, prior to considering any reconstruction and keeping in mind that the biliary tree has only a single arterial supply, is key to performing a vascular assessment. A well-irrigated bile duct is most likely to end up in a successful repair [12] (Fig. 16.4).

On the other hand, AVI conditions a early failure of a bilio-digestive anastomosis (stricture) and greater incidence of bile leaks [13]. Moreover, there is a greater risk of bleeding during biliary repair secondary to the section of arterial collateral circulation of the HP during its dissection, which ultimately exacerbates the ischemia of the biliary tree as we mentioned previously. As a result of this, there is significantly higher morbidity (70 vs. 23%), and mortality observed within uni- and multivariate analysis when an AVI was present at the time of surgical repair (38 vs. 3% when the vasculature was intact). Moreover, recent data reported that AVI ultimately conditioned the indication of reoperations, early and late revascularization, complex liver resections, and even the exceptional consideration for liver transplantation (LT) [14, 15]. Anatomical factors like the proximity of the common bile duct (CBD) to the RHA make this combined injury the most frequent, determining most likely a unilateral hepatic lobe involvement and the higher incidence for right hepatectomies in their ultimate management [16].

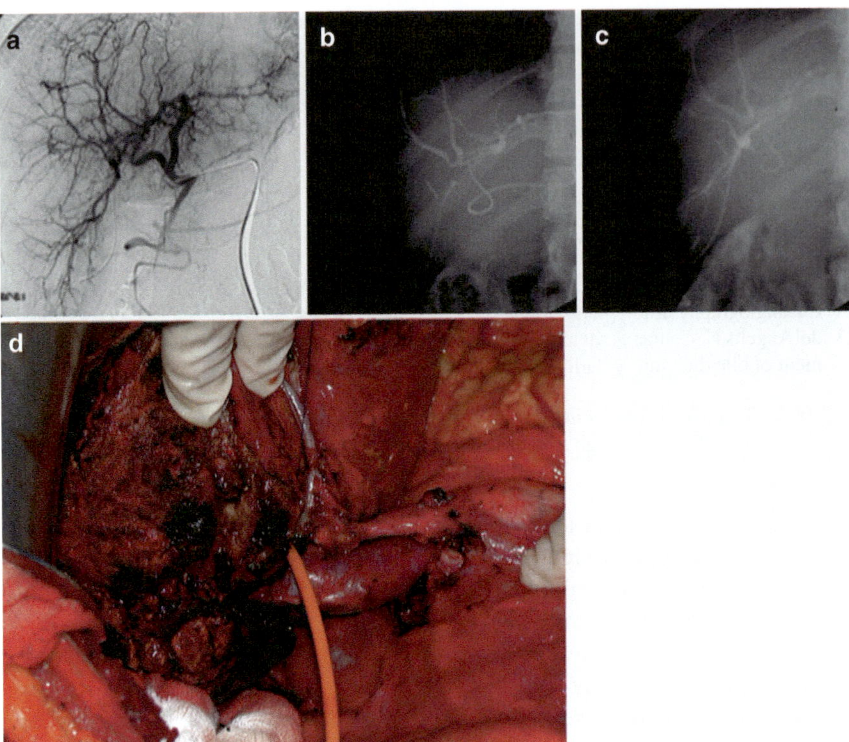

Fig. 16.3 (**a**) Patient with a complex injury involving the right hepatic artery whose right liver is filling through multiple collaterals of the hilar plexus as seen in the angiography. (**b**) Sinusography that confirms the BDI compromised the biliary confluence (absence of visualization of the right hepatic duct). (**c**) The right hepatic duct was visualized when punctured separately. (**d**) The patient was offered a right hepatectomy. An orange catheter has been introduced in the left hepatic ducts prior to the biliary reconstruction

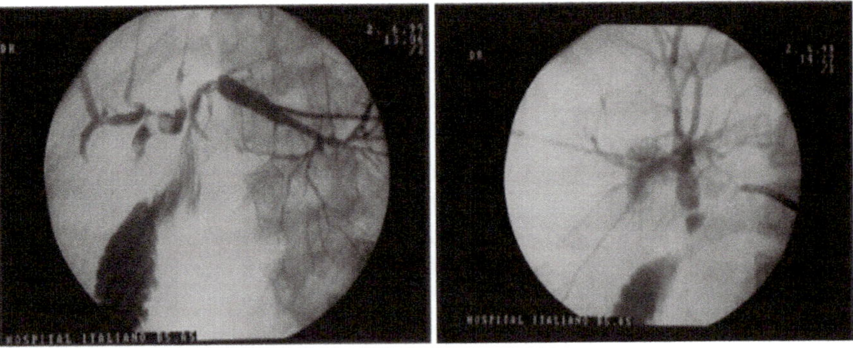

Fig. 16.4 Stricture of a bihepatic-HJ. Given that percutaneous treatment was unsuccessful, a left hepatectomy was performed

In addition, since these injuries usually compromise the RHD, which at the same time has a limited extrahepatic portion, when it suffers an ischemic or thermal injury it can quickly spread towards the proximal biliary tree and may compromise the biliary confluence, leading to a more problematical situation [16].

In the complex scenarios of a BDI with AVI, where the portal circulation is reduced as well, the risk of hepatic necrosis is high and arterial reconstruction should be seriously considered [17].

The overall recommendation in these cases is to proceed with the vascular repair whenever possible and when there is enough experience in vascular surgery to avoid causing further local damage. In early reoperations, the finding of the distal arterial end enables revascularization using preferentially autologous grafts if possible [18, 19].

The mentioned factors related to the type and complexity of the injury, in addition to those related to the patient, and the previous therapies that were offered can determine the appearance of sectorial IC, recurrent cholangitis, liver abscess, recurrent bacteremias, intrahepatic stones, or other septic complications involving one or more segments of the liver [20]. In these circumstances, most of the conservative approaches to restore the liver and biliary function have or are destined to be ineffective and the final solution consists of removing the affected liver lobe or segments [21] (Fig. 16.5a, b).

A liver resection will usually involve the affected liver segments and a Roux-en-Y Hepaticojejunostomy (HJ) reconstruction at the preserved and well-vascularized portion of the biliary tree [22]. This must be comprehensively planned on an elective basis, which means a "cooled down" patient [23]. That is to say, a patient in acceptable general condition, well-nourished, free of cholangitis, and within the appropriate time frame after the injury [12] (Figs. 16.6a, b and 16.7) (See Chap. 11: *Postoperative treatment*).

Several authors have conducted resections within days of injury for the management of complications associated with RPD injuries (leaks) or portal vein branches

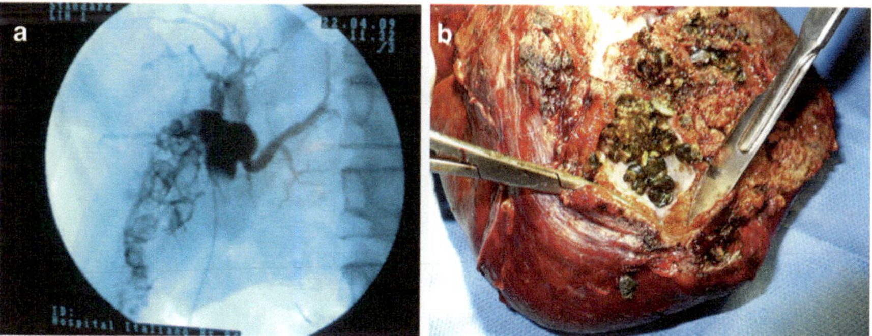

Fig. 16.5 (**a**) Intrahepatic biliary stenosis associated with extensive intrahepatic lithiasis. (**b**) After a right hepatectomy was performed, upon opening the bile duct of the specimen, numerous intrahepatic stones were observed

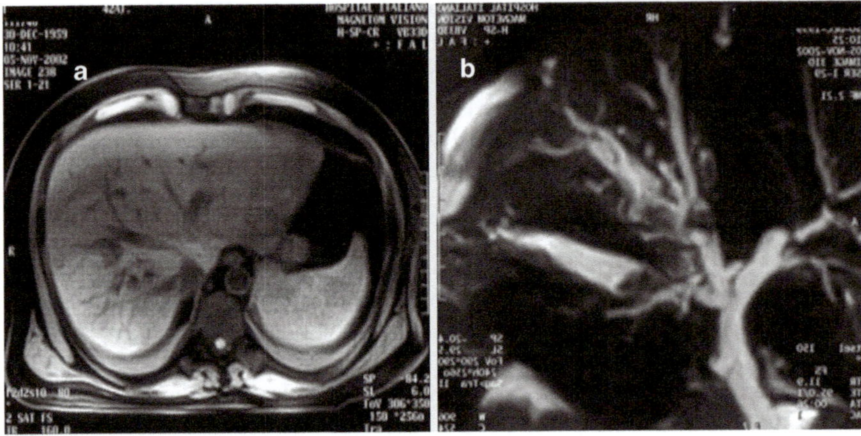

Fig. 16.6 (**a**, **b**) Extensive stricture of the right hepatic ducts associated with right hepatic artery injury. This patient underwent right hepatectomy. A right atrophy and left hypertrophy can be appreciated as well

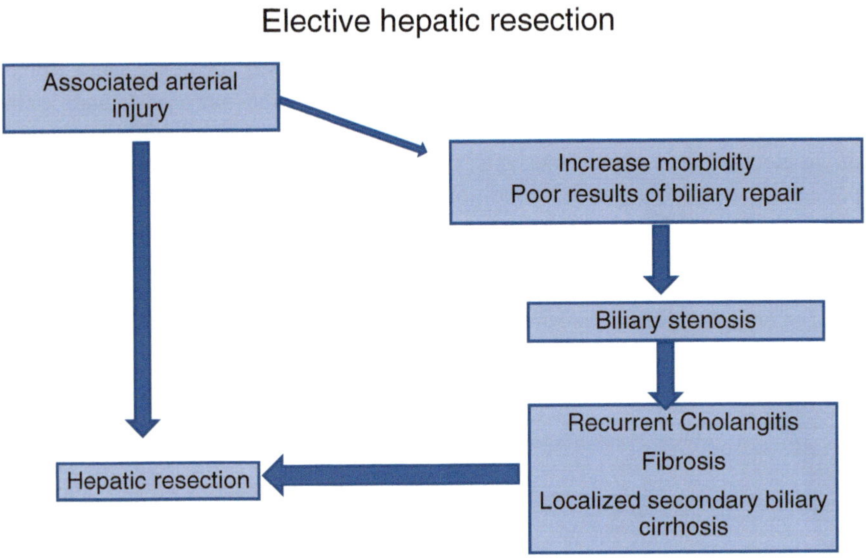

Elective hepatic resection

Associated arterial injury

Increase morbidity
Poor results of biliary repair

Biliary stenosis

Recurrent Cholangitis
Fibrosis
Localized secondary biliary cirrhosis

Hepatic resection

Fig. 16.7 Elective liver resections for arterial injury. Primary or secondary indication after torpid evolution

(hepatic necrosis). However, LR in the acute setting has been associated with high morbidity and mortality and should be contemporized whenever possible [24] (Figs. 16.8 and 16.9).

(*The workup of vascular structures in the context of a BDI are thoroughly explained in Chaps. 9 and 10*)

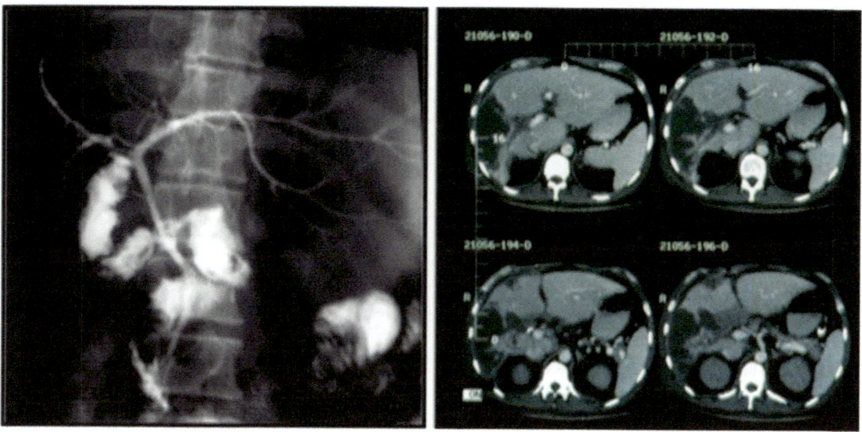

Fig. 16.8 Cholangiogram (left) showing a bile leak from an injury affecting the right posterior duct (RPD). CT scan (right) demonstrated in the same case a concomitant vascular injury in the right posterior pedicle, causing ischemia/necrosis of the right posterior liver segments

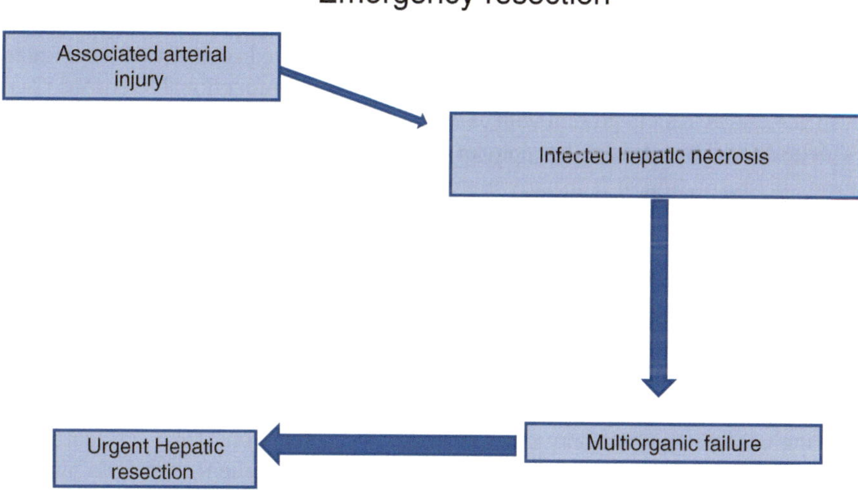

Fig. 16.9 Indications for liver resection in the acute setting

LR Without Underlying AVI

Extensive strictures of the biliary tree, like the ones observed in thermal injuries and/or with AVI, can determine a long course of impaired bile flow, biliary hypertension, and chronic inflammation. If the stricture is insufficiently treated and persists over time, or if IC is already established, it can lead to irreversible changes in the liver parenchyma such as progressive fibrosis and ultimately secondary

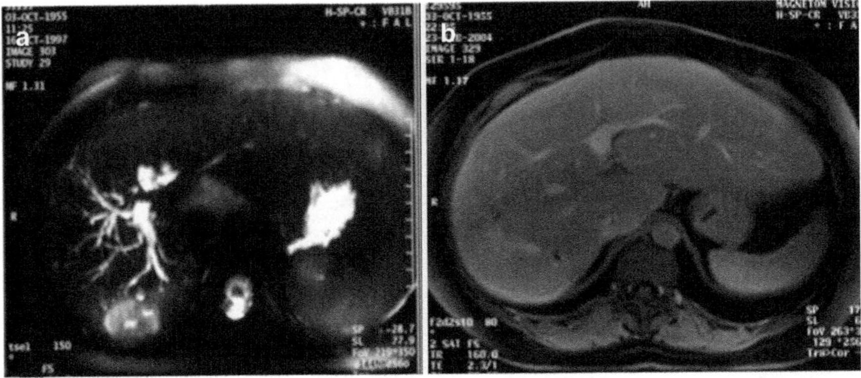

Fig. 16.10 (**a**, **b**) MRI demonstrating a right hepatic duct stricture with upstream dilatation and leading to parenchymal atrophy 4 years after a BDI. This case required a right hepatectomy for recurrent cholangitis

biliary cirrhosis (SBC) [25]. If this affected both hepatic ducts, the best strategy to restore the bile flow should be discussed and the patient should be assessed for liver transplant [26].

However, when this obstruction and cholestasis involves only one of the principal bile ducts, it will determine atrophy of just the affected segment with contralateral hypertrophy of the non-compromised and otherwise functional liver lobe [21].

These cases usually present with extensive stricture on one side of the biliary tree, with upstream dilatation and atrophy of the respective liver lobe (Fig. 16.10a, b). For their final resolution, it is usually more straightforward to proceed with the LR of these hepatic segments/lobe rather than repeated more conservative approaches [27].

Surgical repair of intrahepatic strictures has a high rate of restenosis and recurrent cholangitis (50%), making these cases better and more cost-effective for resolution by LR when the injury is extensive, or by percutaneous treatment when the stricture is limited [28].

In our center, LR for BDI represented 0.8% of all our LR and was needed in only 5% of our patients referred with a BDI. However, they were extremely useful for solving complex cases where other percutaneous, endoscopic, and surgical therapeutic procedures had already failed. The results were excellent, even if technically complex [21, 22, 29].

Most patients with bile duct injuries are young, socially active, many of them disabled after injuries with long-term convalescence due to multiple treatments, and very optimistic about achieving a complete resolution of their problem and improving their quality of life [30].

LR including the injured intrahepatic duct would keep us away from the unsatisfactory high anastomosis with the necessity of prolonged follow-up, reducing long-term complications such as restenosis and recurrent cholangitis. For all these considerations, LR in experienced centers should be considered for the treatment of patients with acceptable operative risk and with high BDI, occasionally with concomitant AVI [31].

Conclusions

Liver resections are rarely applied procedures in the management of BDIs. However, they constitute an excellent alternative in the treatment of complex BDI, especially when there is a destruction of the BC and AVI, or with extended intrahepatic stenosis and/or concomitant lobar atrophy.

A careful patient and case selection are determinant, and the fact that these are technically challenging procedures as a result of sclerosis and inflammation at the porta hepatis, severe adhesions, and the phenomenon of atrophy-hypertrophy of the liver has to be weighed as well.

References

1. Li J, Frilling A, Nadalin S, Broelsch CE, Malago M. Timing and risk factors of hepatectomy in the management of complications following laparoscopic cholecystectomy. J Gastrointest Surg. 2012;16:815–20.
2. Buis CI, Hoekstra H, Verdonk RC, Porte RJ. Causes and consequences of ischemic-type biliary lesions after liver transplantation. J Hepato-Biliary-Pancreat Surg. 2006;13:517–24.
3. Barbier L, Souche R, Slim K, Ah-Soune P. Long-term consequences of bile duct injury after cholecystectomy. J Visc Surg. 2014;151:269–79.
4. Dandekar U, Dandekar K, Chavan S. Right hepatic artery: a cadaver investigation and its clinical significance. Anat Res Int. 2015;2015:412595.
5. Strasberg SM, Helton WS. An analytical review of vasculobiliary injury in laparoscopic and open cholecystectomy. HPB. 2011;13:1–14.
6. Gunji H, Cho A, Tohma T, et al. The blood supply of the hilar bile duct and its relationship to the communicating arcade located between the right and left hepatic arteries. Am J Surg. 2006;192:276–80.
7. Northover JM, Terblanche J. A new look at the arterial supply of the bile duct in man and its surgical implications. Br J Surg. 1979;66:379–84.
8. Plengvanit U, Chearanai O, Sindiivananda K, Damrongsak D, Tuchinda S, Viranuvatti V. Collateral arterial blood supply of the liver after hepatic artery ligation, angiographic study of twenty patients. Ann Surg. 1972;175:105–10.
9. Mercado MA, Domínguez I. Classification and management of bile duct injuries. World J Gastrointest Surg. 2011;3:43–8.
10. Bengmark S, Rosengren K. Angiographic study of the collateral circulation to the liver after ligation of the hepatic artery in man. Am J Surg. 1970;119:620–4.
11. Schmidt SC, Settmacher U, Langrehr JM, Neuhaus P. Management and outcome of patients with combined bile duct and hepatic arterial injuries after laparoscopic cholecystectomy. Surgery. 2004;135:613–8.
12. de'Angelis N, Catena F, Memeo R, et al. 2020 WSES guidelines for the detection and management of bile duct injury during cholecystectomy. World J Emerg Surg. 2021;16:30.

13. Koffron A, Ferrario M, Parsons W, Nemcek A, Saker M, Abecassis M. Failed primary management of iatrogenic biliary injury: incidence and significance of concomitant hepatic arterial disruption. Surgery. 2001;130:722–8. discussion 728–31
14. Pulitanò C, Parks RW, Ireland H, Wigmore SJ, Garden OJ. Impact of concomitant arterial injury on the outcome of laparoscopic bile duct injury. Am J Surg. 2011;201:238–44.
15. Thomson BNJ, Parks RW, Madhavan KK, Garden OJ. Liver resection and transplantation in the management of iatrogenic biliary injury. World J Surg. 2007;31:2363–9.
16. Gupta N, Solomon H, Fairchild R, Kaminski DL. Management and outcome of patients with combined bile duct and hepatic artery injuries. Arch Surg. 1998;133:176–81.
17. Wachsberg RH, Cho KC, Raina S. Liver infarction following unrecognized right hepatic artery ligation at laparoscopic cholecystectomy. Abdom Imaging. 1994;19:53–4.
18. Buell JF, Cronin DC, Funaki B, Koffron A, Yoshida A, Lo A, Leef J, Millis JM. Devastating and fatal complications associated with combined vascular and bile duct injuries during cholecystectomy. Arch Surg. 2002;137:703–8. discussion 708–10
19. Gupta V, Gupta V, Joshi P, Kumar S, Kulkarni R, Chopra N, Pavankumar G, Chandra A. Management of post cholecystectomy vascular injuries. Surgeon. 2019;17:326–33.
20. Walsh RM, Matthew Walsh R, Michael Henderson J, Vogt DP, Brown N. Long-term outcome of biliary reconstruction for bile duct injuries from laparoscopic cholecystectomies. Surgery. 2007;142:450–7.
21. De Santibáñes E, Ardiles V, Pekolj J. Complex bile duct injuries: management. HPB. 2008;10:4–12.
22. Pekolj J, Yanzón A, Dietrich A, del Valle G, Ardiles V, de Santibañes E. Major liver resection as definitive treatment in post-cholecystectomy common bile duct injuries. World J Surg. 2015;39:1216–23.
23. Booij KAC, Coelen RJ, de Reuver PR, Besselink MG, van Delden OM, Rauws EA, Busch OR, van Gulik TM, Gouma DJ. Long-term follow-up and risk factors for strictures after hepaticojejunostomy for bile duct injury: an analysis of surgical and percutaneous treatment in a tertiary center. Surgery. 2018;163:1121–7.
24. Jabłońska B. Hepatectomy for bile duct injuries: when is it necessary? World J Gastroenterol. 2013;19:6348–52.
25. Negi SS, Sakhuja P, Malhotra V, Chaudhary A. Factors predicting advanced hepatic fibrosis in patients with postcholecystectomy bile duct strictures. Arch Surg. 2004;139:299–303.
26. A European-African HepatoPancreatoBiliary Association (E-AHPBA) Research Collaborative Study management group, Other members of the European-African HepatoPancreatoBiliary Association Research Collaborative. Post cholecystectomy bile duct injury: early, intermediate or late repair with hepaticojejunostomy—an E-AHPBA multi-center study. HPB. 2019;21:1641–7.
27. Frilling A, Li J, Weber F, Frühauf NR, Engel J, Beckebaum S, Paul A, Zöpf T, Malago M, Broelsch CE. Major bile duct injuries after laparoscopic cholecystectomy: a tertiary center experience. J Gastrointest Surg. 2004;8:679–85.
28. Truant S, Boleslawski E, Lebuffe G, Sergent G, Pruvot F-R. Hepatic resection for post-cholecystectomy bile duct injuries: a literature review. HPB. 2010;12:334–41.
29. Glinka J, Bruballa R, de Santibañes M, Clariá RS, Ardiles V, Mazza OM, Pekolj J, de Santibañes E. Preoperative portal vein embolization followed by right hepatectomy to treat a complex common bile duct injury in a 5-year-old child. World J Pediatr Surg. 2019;2:e000033.
30. Booij KAC, de Reuver PR, van Dieren S, van Delden OM, Rauws EA, Busch OR, van Gulik TM, Gouma DJ. Long-term impact of bile duct injury on morbidity, mortality, quality of life, and work related limitations. Ann Surg. 2018;268:143–50.
31. Mercado MA, Chan C, Salgado-Nesme N, López-Rosales F. Intrahepatic repair of bile duct injuries. A comparative study. J Gastrointest Surg. 2008;12:364–8.

Chapter 17
Liver Transplantation

Juan Glinka, Eduardo de Santibañes, and Victoria Ardiles

A Bile Duct Injury is like a type of cancer that can be iatrogenically introduced in a patient.

Dr. E. Beveraggi

Introduction

BDI can occur as consequence of any surgical procedure performed in the abdomen. However, laparoscopic cholecystectomy (LC) remains the main accountable one, given not only the frequency in which this procedure is performed but also its vicinity with the porta hepatis (PH). In addition, several factors can distort the anatomy causing confusion and fertile terrain for the development of a BDI [1].

When a BDI occurs, it is associated with high morbidity, higher mortality, a reduced Quality of Life (QoL), and long-term survival. Moreover, this prevails in young patients who have undergone surgery for an otherwise benign condition [2].

A large percentage of BDI is non-adverted during the primary surgery, conditioning a vague postoperative course, that ultimately reduces the chances of immediate restorative treatment.

J. Glinka
Division of HPB Surgery and Multiorgan Transplant Unit, Western University – London Regional Cancer Program, London, ON, Canada

E. de Santibañes · V. Ardiles (✉)
HPB Surgery and Liver Transplant Unit, Hospital Italiano de Buenos Aires, Buenos Aires, Argentina

J. Pekolj et al. (eds.), *Fundamentals of Bile Duct Injuries*, https://doi.org/10.1007/978-3-031-13383-1_17

Therapeutic options for a patient with BDI range from minimally invasive (percutaneous or endoscopic) to surgical management, where biliodigestive shunts and/or liver resections hepatectomies serve as possible alternatives [3].

The aim of any intervention should be focused on restoring the continuity of biliary flow and preventing short- and long-term complications, such as abdominal abscesses, biliary strictures, recurrent cholangitis, and secondary biliary cirrhosis (SBC) [4].

It is not unfrequent to receive a patient that underwent multiple unsuccessful interventions like drains, endoscopic procedures, and reoperations, that hereafter complicate the situation.

This delay in referral to a specialized center to receive definitive and effective treatment not only increases the morbidity but also the likelihood of developing long-term and irreversible complications, such as portal hypertension (PHT) and SBC [5] (Fig. 17.1).

Liver transplantation (LT) constitutes the last option in patients in whom the therapeutic tools to preserve liver function have been exhausted and when irreversible chronic liver disease is already established.

Historical series describe that approximately 10% of patients with BDI repairs ended up developing SBC and death from their related complications when LT is non-feasible [6].

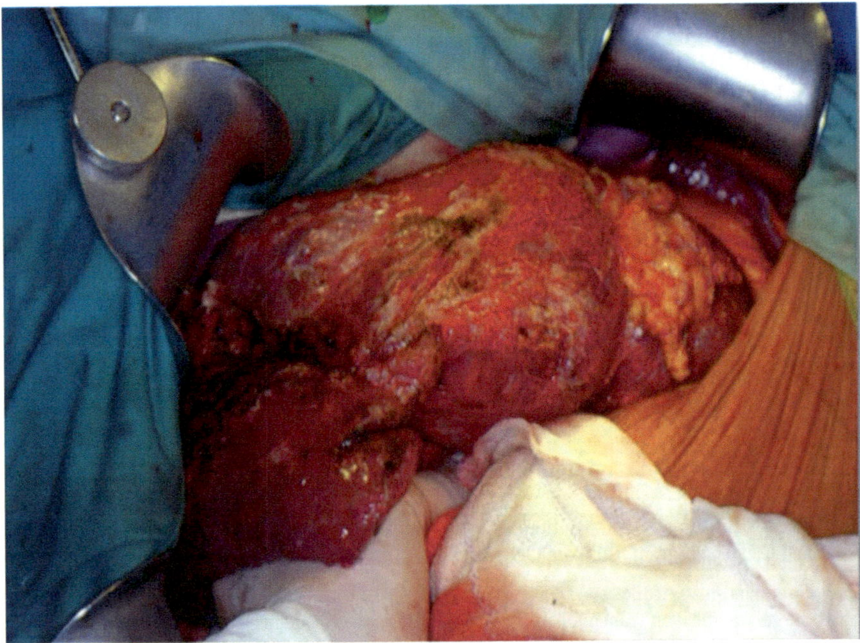

Fig. 17.1 Intraoperative inspection of the liver with SBC due to BDI before starting the hepatectomy for LT

In more recent series, between 3 and 20% of patients with complex BDI have been added to the waiting list for LT as the only possible treatment for their advanced disease.

LT consists of the total removal of the patient's diseased liver and the partial or total implantation of a liver from a living or cadaveric donor. The most used technique is *orthotopic transplantation*. That is to say, removing completely the patient's native liver, and placing a donor's liver (allograft) in its original position (right subphrenic space).

In this population, the use of living donor liver grafts is possible although controversial [7].

Clinical Presentation

There are *two possible scenarios* among patients with BDI who will require LT.

- Patients who develop acute liver failure (ALF) secondary to liver ischemia/necrosis as a result of a BDI along with vascular injury. Because of this catastrophic yet unusual complication, the patient will be placed on the transplant waiting list as an emergency [8].

  Any patient with ALF has already high mortality rates. However, even if the LT is successful these conditions sustain very high mortality in the postoperative period.
- Patients with a BDI develop progressive liver fibrosis and ultimately SBC in the long term. This presentation is, fortunately, more frequent, and the admission to the transplant waiting list is elective [9].

Pathogenesis of End-Stage Liver Disease Due to BDIs

SBC evolves from a gradual and steady process determined by an inadequate biliary outflow. In addition, repeated episodes of cholangitis determine a progressive and irreversible remodelation of the hepatic parenchyma towards fibrosis. This will not only affect the normal liver synthetic function but also may carry systemic complications [10].

Most of the histological changes produced at the onset of obstruction are reversible if treatment is initiated opportunity.

However, patients are often held up in the institution where the BDI was initiated and only referred to specialized centers after multiple ineffective therapies had been ventured, exhibiting signs and symptoms of advanced liver disease [11] (Fig. 17.2).

Several studies correlate the duration of biliary obstruction to the degree of the portal and periportal fibrosis. Such fibrosis usually begins around 3 months after the biliary obstruction commenced, reaching severe levels at 22 months [12].

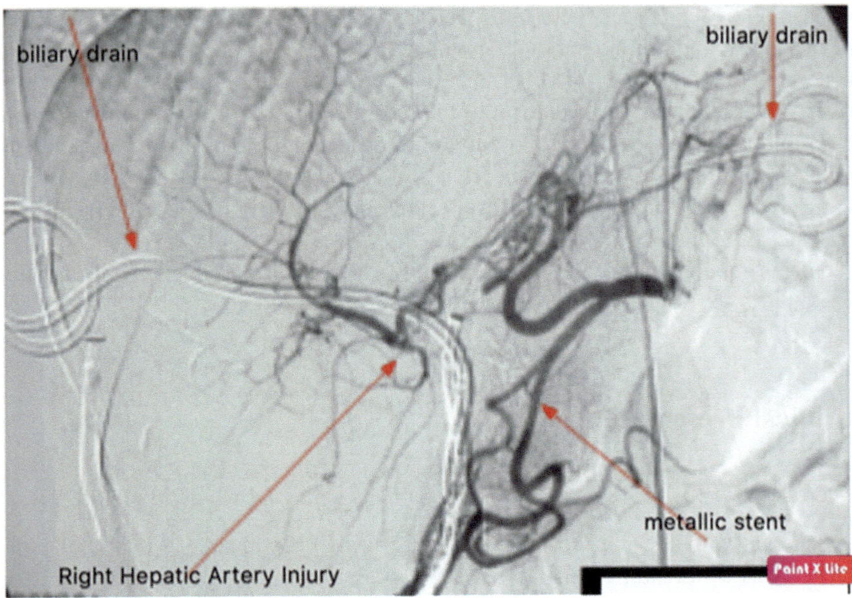

Fig. 17.2 Digital angiography demonstrating the collateral circulation of the hilar plexus developed from left to right as a result of thrombosis of the right hepatic artery (RHA). This patient received multiple treatments that can be appreciated: endoscopic biliary metallic stent, bilateral percutaneous bile duct drains

Irreversible liver cirrhosis takes an average of 62 months to become fully established (Fig. 17.3). The importance of this gradualness underscores the need for an opportune and effective resolution in referral centers before the damage becomes irreversible [13].

Even in advanced stages, cirrhosis does not constitute the worst scenario of end-stage liver disease (ESLD) until portal hypertension (PHT) sets in. The latter is triggered by the presence of marked hepatic fibrosis—cirrhotic stage—, with the consequent resistance in the hepatocellular microcirculation, aggravated by hepatocyte hyperplasia [14].

Its presence constitutes an independent prognostic factor with an overall mortality rate of 26% when these patients undergo a surgical procedure (in contrast to 2% in the absence of PHT). Therefore, these patients' management is considerably more complex and aggressive definitive treatment should be ensured before fibrosis sets in motion [15].

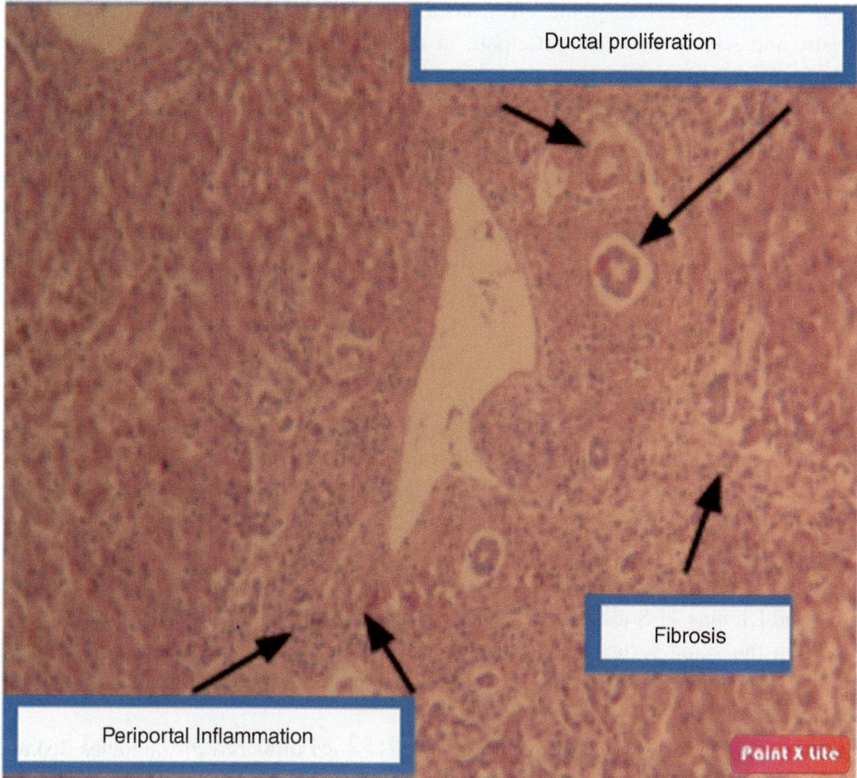

Fig. 17.3 Histological section (Hematoxylin & Eosin stain, 100×) of the liver with canalicular hypertension along with different elements of hepatocellular damage. Portal inflammation, fibroblast proliferation, ductular proliferation, and mononuclear inflammatory infiltrate

Impact of the Problem

The indication for LT in BDIs has declined in recent years, from 3.1% of the LT performed in Argentina from 1990 to 1994 to 0.2% from 2005 to 2010. This probably reflects a better understanding of the pathology, prevention, and more appropriate management, referrals, and multidisciplinary approach to complications [16].

Patient Selection

The primary indication for LT in a patient with BDI is otherwise untreatable ESLD. The need for transplantation, and the inclusion of the patient in a waiting list, is determined on a multidisciplinary basis where transplant surgeons, hepatologists, gastroenterologists, transplant infectious diseases specialists, dietitians, physiotherapists, and social workers participate in the discussion of every potential candidate for LT.

The most common scoring system to rank patients within LT waiting lists is the MELD (Model for End-Stage Liver Disease)—sodium score, which takes biochemical parameters such as bilirubin, International Normalized Ratio (INR), creatinine, and sodium [17].

This scoring system is unfortunately not always fair with patients suffering ESLD secondary to these being conditions since complications such as intractable ascites, progressive jaundice, recurrent variceal hemorrhage, cholangitis, intractable pruritus, and poor QoL do not impact the score as much. As a result, these patients stay longer on the waiting list and arrive at the transplant very deteriorated, or they even die during the time on the waiting list without access to a LT [18].

Occasionally, exception points can be granted upon special requests on a case-by-case basis by the regional Organ Procurement and Transplantation Network.

In a publication by our group, we reported that 3–20% of patients with complex BDI required a LT, representing 7.35% of all transplant recipients from our institution.

In the same report, we observed that the mean time between the generation of the BDI and LT was 41.8 months, with a meantime on the waiting list of 15 months.

From the same series, most patients were included electively, and waiting list mortality has been 22% due to septic or hemorrhagic complications secondary to PHT.

Nevertheless, survival rates were excellent: 92, 81, and 75% at 1, 3, and 5 years of follow-up, respectively [19].

Parrilla et al. published the results of the *Spanish Liver Transplantation Study Group*, in which they reviewed the indications and evolution of 27 patients with postcholecystectomy BDIs who were listed for LT over a period of 24 years.

Seven patients were admitted to the emergency list shortly after a LC, of whom two died on the WL. One of the fatalities was related to sepsis, and the second one corresponding to a patient that remained anhepatic for a prolonged time after total hepatectomy due to massive hepatic necrosis. Four out of five patients who required a LT in emergency conditions died within the first 30 days of the postoperative period.

The remaining 20 patients were admitted under elective conditions for SBC. In this subgroup, 5-year survival reached 68%, which is ultimately lower than survival expected for LT for other causes [20].

Table 17.1 describes the main reports of LT in the treatment of BDIs.

Table 17.1 Historical series reporting liver transplantation as a treatment for complications of bile duct injuries

Author	Year	*N*	Primary procedure	Reason of LD	Postoperative mortality
Bacha et al. [21]	1994	1	LC	FLF	No
Robertson et al. [22]	1998	1	LC	SBC	No
Loinaz et al. [23]	2001	12	7 EGCR, 4 CC, 1 RH	SBC	1/12 patients
Nordin et al. [5]	2002	5	4 LC, 1 CC	SBC	1/5 patients
Fernandez et al. [24]	2004	2	LC	FLF	2/2 patients
Oncel et al. [25]	2006	1	CC	SBC	No
Thompson et al. [26]	2007	2	CC	SBC	1/2 patients
deSantibanañes et al. [19]	2008	16	10 CC, 3 LC, 1 RH, 2 EGCR	SBC	2/16 patients
Zaydfudim et al. [27]	2009	2	1 LC, 1 Adrenalectomy	FLF	No
Mc Cormack et al. [8]	2009	1	LC	FLF	1/1 patients
Ardiles et al. [16]	2010	19	10 CC, 6 LC, 1 RH, 2 EGCR	SBC y 1 FLF	4/8 patients
Parilla et al. [20]	2013	27	13 CC, 14 LC	5 FLF, 20 SBC	5/27 patients
Leale et al. [28]	2016	3	CC 1, LC 1	1 FLF, 2 SBC	No

LC Laparoscopic Cholecystectomy, *CC* Conventional Cholecystectomy, *EGCR* Echinococcus Cysts Resection, *RH* Right Hepatectomy, *FLF* Fulminant Liver Failure, *SBC* Secondary Biliary Cirrhosis

Prognosis

LT in patients with BDIs is technically more complex because of adhesions due to multiple previous surgeries, fibrosis, and inflammation throughout the PH, coagulopathy, PHT, atrophy-hypertrophy phenomenon, and septic complications.

Long-term survival in LT patients is slightly lower than that of patients undergoing a LT for BDIs. In addition, the perioperative morbidity and mortality seem higher than the reported for SBC and other etiologies [29].

Prevention

Correct management of patients with BDI is essential to ensure long-term survival. Multiple failed interventions by inexperienced teams and delays in referral to specialized centers are directly related to late, severe, and irreversible complications in BDIs.

SBC and PHT cause significant morbimortality, requiring LT as the only possible treatment. LT is usually difficult and with significant postoperative morbidity. Although it provides long-term survival with acceptable QoL, it still represents a high biological cost for a patient that initially underwent a routine surgical procedure for the treatment of benign disease.

References

1. Jabłońska B, Lampe P. Iatrogenic bile duct injuries: etiology, diagnosis and management. World J Gastroenterol. 2009;15:4097–104.
2. Booij KAC, de Reuver PR, van Dieren S, van Delden OM, Rauws EA, Busch OR, van Gulik TM, Gouma DJ. Long-term impact of bile duct injury on morbidity, mortality, quality of life, and work related limitations. Ann Surg. 2018;268:143–50.
3. de'Angelis N, Catena F, Memeo R, et al. 2020 WSES guidelines for the detection and management of bile duct injury during cholecystectomy. World J Emerg Surg. 2021;16:30.
4. Guieu M, Chiche L, Bachelier P, et al. Liver transplantation for iatrogenic bile duct injury during cholecystectomy: French retrospective multicentric study. HPB. 2020;22:S333–4.
5. Nordin A, Halme L, Mäkisalo H, Isoniemi H, Höckerstedt K. Management and outcome of major bile duct injuries after laparoscopic cholecystectomy: from therapeutic endoscopy to liver transplantation. Liver Transpl. 2002;8:1036–43.
6. Barbier L, Souche R, Slim K, Ah-Soune P. Long-term consequences of bile duct injury after cholecystectomy. J Visc Surg. 2014;151:269–79.
7. Rossi M, Mennini G, Lai Q, Ginanni Corradini S, Drudi FM, Pugliese F, Berloco PB. Liver transplantation. J Ultrasound. 2007;10:28–45.
8. McCormack L, Quiñonez EG, Capitanich P, Chao S, Serafini V, Goldaracena N, Mastai RC. Acute liver failure due to concomitant arterial, portal and biliary injury during laparoscopic cholecystectomy: is transplantation a valid life-saving strategy? A case report. Patient Saf Surg. 2009;3:22.
9. Vilatoba M, Chavez-Villa M, Figueroa-Mendez R, Dominguez-Rosado I, Cruz-Martinez R, Leal-Villalpando RP, Garcia-Juarez I, Mercado MA. Liver transplantation as definitive treatment of post-cholecystectomy bile duct injury: experience in a high-volume repair center. Ann Surg. 2021; https://doi.org/10.1097/SLA.0000000000005245.
10. Pinzani M, Luong TV. Pathogenesis of biliary fibrosis. Biochim Biophys Acta Mol basis Dis. 2018;1864:1279–83.
11. Patrono D, Benvenga R, Colli F, Baroffio P, Romagnoli R, Salizzoni M. Surgical management of post-cholecystectomy bile duct injuries: referral patterns and factors influencing early and long-term outcome. Updat Surg. 2015;67:283–91.
12. Tag CG, Sauer-Lehnen S, Weiskirchen S, Borkham-Kamphorst E, Tolba RH, Tacke F, Weiskirchen R. Bile duct ligation in mice: induction of inflammatory liver injury and fibrosis by obstructive cholestasis. J Vis Exp. 2015; https://doi.org/10.3791/52438.
13. Schreuder AM, Busch OR, Besselink MG, Ignatavicius P, Gulbinas A, Barauskas G, Gouma DJ, van Gulik TM. Long-term impact of iatrogenic bile duct injury. Dig Surg. 2020;37:10–21.
14. Iwakiri Y. Pathophysiology of portal hypertension. Clin Liver Dis. 2014;18:281–91.
15. Wong M, Busuttil RW. Surgery in patients with portal hypertension. Clin Liver Dis. 2019;23:755–80.
16. Ardiles V, McCormack L, Quiñonez E, Goldaracena N, Mattera J, Pekolj J, Ciardullo M, de Santibañes E. Experience using liver transplantation for the treatment of severe bile duct injuries over 20 years in Argentina: results from a National Survey. HPB. 2011;13:544–50.
17. de Freitas ACT, Rampim AT, Nunes CP, Coelho JCU. Impact of meld sodium on liver transplantation waiting list. Arq Bras Cir Dig. 2019;32:e1460.
18. Tsaparas P, Machairas N, Ardiles V, et al. Liver transplantation as last-resort treatment for patients with bile duct injuries following cholecystectomy: a multicenter analysis. Ann Gastroenterol Hepatol. 2021;34:111–8.
19. de Santibañes E, Ardiles V, Gadano A, Palavecino M, Pekolj J, Ciardullo M. Liver transplantation: the last measure in the treatment of bile duct injuries. World J Surg. 2008;32:1714–21.
20. Parrilla P, Robles R, Varo E, Jiménez C, Sánchez-Cabús S, Pareja E, Spanish Liver Transplantation Study Group. Liver transplantation for bile duct injury after open and laparoscopic cholecystectomy. Br J Surg. 2014;101:63–8.

21. Bacha EA, Stieber AC, Galloway JR, Hunter JG. Non-biliary complication of laparoscopic cholecystectomy. Lancet. 1994;344:896–7.
22. Robertson AJ, Rela M, Karani J, Steger AC, Benjamin IS, Heaton ND. Laparoscopic cholecystectomy injury: an unusual indication for liver transplantation. Transpl Int. 1998;11:449–51.
23. Loinaz C, González EM, Jiménez C, García I, Gómez R, González-Pinto I, Colina F, Gimeno A. Long-term biliary complications after liver surgery leading to liver transplantation. World J Surg. 2001;25:1260–3.
24. Fernández JA, Robles R, Marín C, Sánchez-Bueno F, Ramírez P, Parrilla P. Laparoscopic iatrogeny of the hepatic hilum as an indication for liver transplantation. Liver Transpl. 2004;10:147–52.
25. Oncel D, Ozden I, Bilge O, Tekant Y, Acarli K, Alper A, Emre A, Arioğul O. Bile duct injury during cholecystectomy requiring delayed liver transplantation: a case report and literature review. Tohoku J Exp Med. 2006;209:355–9.
26. Thomson BNJ, Parks RW, Madhavan KK, Garden OJ. Liver resection and transplantation in the management of iatrogenic biliary injury. World J Surg. 2007;31:2363–9.
27. Zaydfudim V, Wright JK, Pinson CW. Liver transplantation for iatrogenic porta hepatis transection. Am Surg. 2009;75:313–6.
28. Leale I, Moraglia E, Bottino G, Rachef M, Dova L, Cariati A, De Negri A, Diviacco P, Andorno E. Role of liver transplantation in bilio-vascular liver injury after cholecystectomy. Transplant Proc. 2016;48:370–6.
29. Addeo P, Saouli A-C, Ellero B, Woehl-Jaegle M-L, Oussoultzoglou E, Rosso E, Cesaretti M, Bachellier P. Liver transplantation for iatrogenic bile duct injuries sustained during cholecystectomy. Hepatol Int. 2013;7:910–5.

Index

J. Pekolj et al. (eds.), *Fundamentals of Bile Duct Injuries*,
https://doi.org/10.1007/978-3-031-13383-1

GPSR Compliance

The European Union's (EU) General Product Safety Regulation (GPSR) is a set of rules that requires consumer products to be safe and our obligations to ensure this.

If you have any concerns about our products, you can contact us on ProductSafety@springernature.com

In case Publisher is established outside the EU, the EU authorized representative is:

Springer Nature Customer Service Center GmbH
Europaplatz 3
69115 Heidelberg, Germany

Batch number: 09755383

Printed by Printforce, the Netherlands